DOCUMENTING FUNCTION
PHYSICAL THERAPY

Documenting Functional Outcomes in Physical Therapy

DARLENE L. STEWART, M.S., P.T.
Professor and Chair
Physical Therapy Department
California State University, Fresno
Fresno, California

SUSAN H. ABELN, P.T., A.R.M.
President
Strategic Healthcare Alternative
San Clemente, California

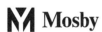 Mosby

St. Louis Baltimore Boston Chicago London Philadelphia Sydney Toronto

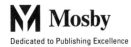

Mosby
Dedicated to Publishing Excellence

Sponsoring Editor: David K. Marshall/Martha Sasser
Project Supervisor, Text and Reference: George Mary Gardner
Project Supervisor: Carol A. Reynolds
Proofroom Manager: Barbara M. Kelly

2   3   4   5   6   7   8   9   0   CL   MV   97   96   95   94

Library of Congress Cataloging-in-Publication Data
Documenting Functional Outcomes in Physical Therapy
  [edited by] Darlene L. Stewart, Susan H. Abeln.
      p.   cm.
    Includes bibliographical references and index.
    ISBN 0-8016-6359-8
    1. Physical therapy—Practice. 2. Physical therapy—
Documentation.   3. Physical therapy—Decision making.   I. Stewart.
Darlene L.   II. Abeln, Susan H.
    [DNLM: 1. Delivery of Health Care—organization & administration.
2. Medical Records. 3. Physical Therapy.   4. Reimbursement
Mechanisms—organization & administration.   WB 460 R425 1993]
RM713.R47   1993
615.8'2'068—dc20
DNLM/DLC
for Library of Congress   92-48392
                                                                            CIP

To my husband, Keith, for his encouragement in creating this work.

Darlene L. Stewart

To my mother and loving husband for their patience and support throughout this project, and to my father for his counsel and tireless effort to bring order out of chaos.

Susan H. Abeln

CONTRIBUTORS

Susan H. Abeln, P.T., A.R.M.
President
Strategic Healthcare Alternative
San Clemente, California

Corinne T. Ellingham, M.S., P.T.
Associate Professor
Program in Physical Therapy
University of Minnesota
Co-Chairman
Minnesota APTA Quality Assurance
Minneapolis, Minnesota

Linda Esposto, P.T.
Executive Director of Personnel
Martin, McCough, and Eddy Physical
  Therapy Services
Pittsburgh, Pennsylvania
Consultant
Allegheny & Chesapeake Physical
  Therapists, Inc.
Johnstown, Pennsylvania

Bette Ann Harris, M.S., P.T.
Director
Graduate Program in Physical Therapy
M.G.H. Institute of Health Professions
Clinical Consultant
Physical Therapy Services
Massachusetts General Hospital
Boston, Massachusetts

Darlene L. Stewart, M.S., P.T.
Professor and Chair
Physical Therapy Department
California State University, Fresno
Fresno, California

Gretchen Swanson, P.T., M.P.H.
President
Swanson & Company
Long Beach, California

FOREWORD

I have followed the events and remarkable changes that have occurred in the delivery and reimbursement of health care in this country for more than 40 years. My interest in this subject has been sustained and intensified because of my involvement in the delivery of physical therapy services and active participation in the affairs of my state and national professional associations throughout this period. Therefore I am delighted to have this opportunity to comment on where physical therapists, as well as other health care professionals, stand today with respect to this complex issue. This text will definitely inform practitioners of what they must do to comply with present and evolving requirements related to this subject.

Health care is widely discussed today, and rarely a day passes that this matter does not attract national attention in the media. The reasons for this widespread coverage should be clear when you consider that health care costs in the United States have increased from $12 billion in 1950 to an estimated $800 billion in 1992, and are projected to reach $1.5 trillion by the year 2000. Per capita health care costs in the United States are higher than in any other industrialized country in the world. Despite our being one of the richest countries, some 60 million people are either unisured or marginally insured. Some 20% to 30% of all medical procedures performed in this country, and which cost the system about $125 billion a year, may not be warranted. Furthermore, about 20% of all health care expenditures are consumed by administrative costs. Unfortunately, we lack national data to support the comparative results of routinely performed procedures. Very little research has been conducted to determine the effectiveness of our clinical interventions. In fact, Uwe E. Reinhardt, Ph.D., a James Madison Professor of Political Economy from Princeton University and a true scholar of both national and international health policy, sums up the status of the U.S. health care system as lacking in such critical areas as social equity, portability, administrative simplicity, and equity among payers.

Is it any wonder that those responsible for paying these horrendous medical costs are now asserting themselves in a forceful and positive manner in an attempt to bring this system back to some level of normalcy? The remedial efforts taken by third-party payers in the past have not stemmed the tide of health care spending. Each year these costs continue to rise and are outstripping any other sector of the U.S. economy. More drastic measures to curtail what seems to be an insatiable demand for health services have met with finite resources of third-party payers such as government, employers, and patients, who are now being asked to pay an increasing portion of their health care premiums.

For many years physical therapists have been admonished as a profession because of our failure to carry out scientific research to document the efficacy of our services. There can be no question that such research is essential for our profession. However, today we face an equally great challenge that also has the potential to disrupt delivery of our services. I refer specifically to the type of documentation that will demand that we report the results of patient interventions in functional terms. This approach to documentation will be new to many practitioners. Nevertheless, physical therapists and other providers must be well grounded in this system of reporting, to compete in the changing health care industry.

The evolution of our health care system has been chronicled in a comprehensive and organized manner in the opening chapter of this book, and key events that have modified our health care system are identified. This review sets the stage for the remaining chapters, which address many of the contemporary issues related to documentation and outcome reporting.

The reasons why our methods of documentation must change for both governmental and private payers is made abundantly clear in this text. Judging from my experience in reviewing physical therapy claims, proper documentation on which rational decisions concerning reimbursement can be made is sadly lacking in our profession. The longevity of any practice may well hinge on the practitioner's ability to clearly describe the effectiveness of interventions in quantifiable terms. In the absence of such documentation, the likelihood of being reimbursed for the services we provide will indeed be remote.

Of particular interest to all physical therapists will be the chapters describing several approaches to functional outcome reporting and documentation and outcome assessment. There is sufficient evidence that physical therapists and other rehabilitation specialists will have to report and document the services they provide in a manner that truly reflects the functional changes that have occurred as a result of our treatment. I believe this type of reporting is critical to the future vitality of all rehabilitative services. We simply must demonstrate that our interventions can be quantified in functional terms that relate to a patient's impairment and how functional deficits have been modified as a result of treatment.

Third-party payers will not continue to reimburse providers for services whose outcomes are described in vague terms. They will demand precise measurements of progress to justify spending their shrinking health care dollars. I see this as the greatest challenge facing physical therapists today. Conversely, I also see it as an opportunity for us to acquire even greater professional involvement in developing health care programs.

I regret that a text of this type was not available to physical therapists and other health care providers long ago. I am certain that if that had been the case, it would have reduced numerous problems related to the issues addressed in this work. The authors message is clear, and should be self-evident to all who read this text: that is, health care providers, including physical therapists, must understand the importance of how documentation requirements have changed. Those responsible for the task of preparing this text are to be commended for their efforts and for the contribution they have made to all professionals who deliver rehabilitative services.

Charles M. Magistro, P.T., FAPTA

PREFACE

A major priority of Physical Therapists today as they cope with the constraints of managed care is maintaining proficiency in making clinical decisions that demonstrate clearly that their treatment interventions are effective and efficient. As the dollars for health care become less available, payers in the delivery system continue to focus more on concepts of outcome that they are convinced demonstrate that the services they pay for are "reasonable and necessary." They are becoming more convinced that the relationship between treatment intervention and functional outcome must be a priority in their reimbursement decisions. The mechanism for demonstrating such outcomes achieved by the provider is the documentation report.

This text discusses a variety of documentation models that demonstrate the conceptual framework of clinical decision analysis, which is the cornerstone to functional outcome planning and assessment. Examples of appropriate and inappropriate reporting are given, along with the expectations of a variety of payers (private payers, Medicare, Workers Compensation) when making reimbursement decisions based on this documentation.

Case studies demonstrating concepts of functional outcome assessment and reporting also are included, along with sample cases on which readers can practice their own clinical decision and functional outcome reporting skills.

Also discussed is the relationship between patient care and quality assurance in reimbursement issues. An overview of the political and economic indicators that influence the evolution of health care policy in the United States is provided. It is essential that all practitioners understand the delivery environment in which they practice, to be effective participants. As health care policy has moved from a retrospective, unlimited access perspective of health care delivery to managed care with restricted access, providers must be proficient at meeting the rigors of the system.

This reference manual will educate the entry level practitioner in the development and/or refinement of documentation skills, using a functional outcome assessment approach to patient evaluation and treatment intervention. It is intended to assist practitioners in increasing their effectiveness through validation of the efficacy of the physical therapy services.

Darlene L. Stewart, M.S., P.T.
Susan H. Abeln, P.T., A.R.M.

ACKNOWLEDGEMENT

We thank Bette Ann Harris, Gretchen Swanson, Linda Esposto, and Corinne Ellingham for their generosity in sharing their professional expertise in development of this book

Darlene L. Stewart
Susan H. Abeln

CONTENTS

Foreword   *ix*

Preface   *xiii*

1 / Health Care Delivery System   *1*
   by Darlene L. Stewart

2 / Importance of Documentation to Patient Care Reimbursement   *32*
   by Susan H. Abeln

3 / Building Documentation Using a Clinical Decision-Making Model   *81*
   by Bette Ann Harris

4 / Functional Outcome Report: The Next Generation in Physical Therapy
   Reporting   *101*
   by Gretchen Swanson

5 / Applying Functional Outcome Assessment to Medicare Documentation
   135
   by Linda Esposto

6 / Quality Assurance and Total Quality Management   *175*
   by Corinne T. Ellingham and Susan H. Abeln

Glossary   *211*

Appendixes   *221*

Index   *283*

CHAPTER 1

Health Care Delivery System

Darlene L. Stewart, M.S., P.T.

Key Concepts

- Need to understand U.S. health care delivery system
- Coping with a Managed Health Care delivery system
- Purpose of a health care delivery system
- System defects as catalyst for change
- Objectives and strategies of a delivery system
- Evolution of U.S. health care policy
- Future of health care policy

NEED TO UNDERSTAND THE HEALTH CARE DELIVERY SYSTEM

As providers of specialty rehabilitation services, physical therapists often have limited awareness of the intricacies of the delivery system in which they work. This limitation contributes to a lack of understanding of the relationship between the services they provide and the control and distribution of financial resources of health care services in general. Physical therapists often lose sight of the "big picture" as they become intensely involved in their own professional agendas. Consequently they approach their practice without realizing that their priorities may at times be very much different from those of the delivery system. During the past two decades many practitioners have experienced frustration and anxiety as their practice priorities and those of the delivery system have become more divergent.

Persons who pursue the career of Physical Therapist do so with various

1

motivations: Some have a strong altruistic desire to serve others; others are drawn to the profession by a personal interest in some aspect of the profession or because of its financial opportunities. Once the decision has been made to pursue education in the profession, the student's focus, and in many cases the curriculum, often is on acquisition of a knowledge base in clinical science and those clinical skills considered essential for the competent practitioner. As a result of this focus, less attention is usually given to gaining more than a cursory understanding of the elements of the delivery system in which physical therapy services are provided. Opportunities to learn how to implement economic strategies to assure financial stability in practice are often neglected.

Physical Therapist As Provider of Health Care

The most rewarding aspect of being a physical therapist is to help others who are suffering from a dysfunction as a result of disease or injury. However, a new health care environment that focuses on the precept of **managed care** has emerged that places increasing limitations on access to a variety of health care services, including physical therapy services. To assure continued broad access to these services by the public now and in the future, physical therapists have a responsibility not only to be a master clinician but to possess the requisite skills to provide services within the constraints of this altered delivery system. In many cases this means stepping outside the role of clinician and becoming involved in the political and economic processes that influence the policy that directs health care planning. They must learn how to apply economic concepts to demonstrate the value of their services in terms of effectiveness and efficiency. Most important, they must be prepared to demonstrate to the system that physical therapy is an essential service that contributes to the maintenance of optimal health for the population. As resources to finance health care are increasingly curtailed competition by all providers for the health care dollar will be severe. Payer efforts to limit the volume of services available in the system will be linked with a perceived or demonstrated value of the individual service. Such impressions will be evaluated in terms of the total dollars expended for all health care. This point of view will have an impact on all providers, including physical therapists. As acknowledged providers of health care, we cannot practice in a vacuum. We are part of the system and must function within its design, subject to its rules, opportunities, and constraints.

A familiar scenario often occurs as the new graduate, armed with a license, enters practice. Full of enthusiasm and confidence at having reached this career goal, the graduate believes that all things are possible and that his or her professional life holds unlimited opportunities for using expert skills to service the needs of clients referred. It is not surprising that this optimistic naivete is short lived as the new practitioner slowly comes to grips with the realities of practice. After a relatively short time the graduate comes to the conclusion that practicing physical therapy is not what was expected. To some degree, this "reality shock" is experienced by all new workers entering the workplace. When the business aspects of practice are discussed with physical therapists, both the new graduate and the experienced clinician will admit that somewhere during their education someone did mention documentation, reimbursement systems, diagnosis-related groups (DRGs), preferred provider organizations (PPOs), quality assurance processes, health care economics, and the like. However, they did not really think these matters applied to them. After all they did not go into the profession to be involved in the business of it, but to treat patients and give quality care.

In general, this attitude tends to prevail as the graduate becomes socialized into the profession. These attitudes have led us to believe, which some may view as harsh, that many experienced as well as novice practitioners do not see financial management and quality assurance as serious aspects of practice, regardless of the setting. This belief is further reinforced by the priorities that practitioners place on professional growth activities, most of which focus on acquiring or updating of clinical skills. They ignore professional development courses in management, economics, and health care administration. In my opinion, failure to place value on these business skills impairs the practitioner's effectiveness as a professional health care provider.

Despite reforms in health care policy over the past two decades, many, if not most, practitioners continue to hold tenaciously to the philosophy of providing unlimited care to all patients, without serious regard for dollars expended. They insist on this posture even as the delivery system more frequently requires the practitioner to demonstrate that treatment outcome is worth the dollars spent for the services rendered. This incongruence often results in frustration and inability on the part of the practitioner to function effectively within the delivery system. In addition, a multitude of designs used for reimbursement of health care services adds to this frustration, because the practitioner must not only justify the cost of services provided but also determine which of the rules and regulations created by acceptable third-party payers apply to a specific patient. Figure 1–1 is a graphic illustration of how health care is paid for in the United States. It clearly illustrates the complexities of this aspect of practice.

An abundance of information has been disseminated by the media, gov-

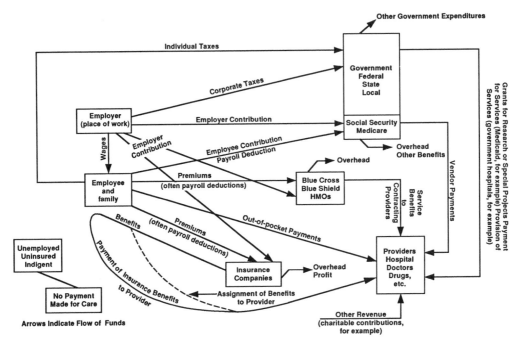

FIG 1–1.
Flow of funds for payment of health care services in the United States. (From Wilson FA, Neuhauser D: *Health Services in the United States.* Cambridge, Mass, 1974, Ballinger Publishing, p 91. Used by permission.)

ernment agencies, and provider groups regarding issues of cost escalation, new concepts of reimbursement, accessibility or inaccessibility of basic health care, and the perceived unmet health care needs of all factions of the U.S. population. As health care providers and planners wrestle with current political and economic health care agendas in response to the public's expectations, all providers can expect to be scrutinized regarding cost effectiveness and efficiency of the services they provide. Today it is not enough to be technically excellent in practice. Health care policy will continue to focus on **competition** as a driving force to lower or decrease cost escalation in the delivery system. The degree to which one succeeds in the system will depend on two factors: the practitioner's ability to compete with other providers for referrals, and how well the principles of economics are applied when making clinical decisions that reflect effective and efficient treatment outcomes. According to Mooney, a world health care economist, the term **economics** means the use of resources to ensure that society gets the best possible return in terms of human welfare from the resources that are available.[2] To a degree, practice success, and in some cases survival, may depend on the practitioner's sophistication in including such concepts in practice and recognizing and responding appropriately to change in the delivery system design. Many practitioners have ignored recent health care policy changes that have altered the traditional delivery system in which we have worked. Many have hoped that these changes would not work, would be ineffective, or would go away. This has not been the case, and is not likely to be so in the future.

During the past 40 years health care providers, especially hospitals and physicians, have been viewed as the major players in the delivery system. They are considered to be the key to its **market dynamics.** Consequently most health planning policy decisions have been targeted at these groups to achieve the health care priorities for the nation. When the system gets out of hand, these groups usually have been the unrelenting target of efforts to control it, especially in the area of cost of health care. In this context, we believe that during the next decade the practitioner will need to direct some attention to four major policy views:

1. Efforts to control the delivery system through hospital inpatient services and the physician provider segments as the target will continue.

2. Efforts to reach out to include most, if not all, outpatient services, regardless of provider setting, will increase.

3. The concepts of **selective pricing** (predetermined fees for specific services) will be the predominant means of rationing or controlling access and volume of all health care services. Modified versions of existing **prospective payment** concepts (DRGs) will gain support for inclusion in outpatient as well as inpatient service areas.

4. Consumers will continue to be pressed to make choices regarding the amount and type of health care services they are willing to pay for as payers (both government and private) increase efforts to abdicate financial risk of paying for health care to business, labor, and the individual household.

These policy views will create added financial risk for physical therapists. They especially will have an impact on providers in outpatient settings or private practice who rely heavily on private insurers as opposed to government and the individual for the bulk of their reimbursement. An integral part of managing this financial risk will be the use of **quality assurance** processes and utilization review. The review and quality assurance processes will focus on measurement of treatment outcomes. This measurement will determine appropriateness of care and form the basis for reimbursement decisions as policy makers and insurers remain unconvinced that *all care given is medically necessary.* The vehicle for review will be patient care documentation. The admonitions that "If it does not appear in writing, it did not occur," and "If it is not functional, it is not relevant" will continue to be heard.

The purpose of this book is to provide physical therapists with the tools to improve or modify clinical decision making and documentation skills to enhance effectiveness in using **outcome assessment** concepts as a tool for reimbursement. We first explore major events and factors of the past that have influenced the way health care services are accessed and delivered. Second, we discuss what we believe will be future health care reforms.

COPING WITH MANAGED HEALTH CARE DELIVERY SYSTEM

The delivery system in which we practice is complex and multidimensional. An in-depth description of these dimensions is certainly beyond the scope of this book. Our intent is to present, through the perspectives of a number of leading health care analysts and researchers, a sense of the political and economic events and factors that have been catalysts for the evolution of a new health care delivery system design, managed care, especially as it relates to reimbursement. This brief commentary is intended to enlighten you and to effect a positive change in your attitude about the system. It will improve your understanding about how health care policy is set, and describe internal and external factors that influence policy change, so that you can more effectively plan for your practice needs. Effectiveness in responding to change requires, at a minimum, an understanding of the nuances of the health care delivery system in the United States and cognizance of the specific events that have influenced change in the system over the past five decades. The effective practitioner understands the past, current, and future philosophies and agendas of health care policy and is prepared to implement new approaches to delivery of care that are in concert with policy. Most important, he or she is open to and willing to make timely changes in practice to respond to the dictates of the system. In contrast, the practitioner who clings to the old way of doing things may fall by the wayside. There is little doubt that the competition for the health care dollar will become more acute as health care resources continue to shrink. Those who possess political acuity and who manage their practices in an efficient and cost-effective manner based on sound economic principles, within the dictates of the system, will be successful.

Cause of Escalation of Health Care Costs

According to most health care policy analysts, three major factors over the past 40 years have led to the current problem of excessive health care costs: increased access to services, greater population, and expanded technology. A fourth factor, identified more recently (1975–1985), is general inflation and the aging of the U.S. population.[2] Another factor mentioned less frequently in the literature, but which underlies the concept of market incentives, is the tendency by consumers and providers to overuse or consume large volumes of services in the system. In more recent years the inability or reluctance of politicians, special interest groups, and labor and industry to come to agreement on solutions to system **design defects** has also contributed to the problem. Another factor that should not be overlooked is the expectation of the citizenry that health care, regardless of cost, is a right rather than a privilege. Society expects access to all levels and unlimited amounts of health care regardless of ability to pay for that care. This philosophy pervades all deliberations in the modification of health care policy. This philosophy, however, is not necessarily shared by government and business, which pay for most health care today.

PURPOSE OF A HEALTH CARE DELIVERY SYSTEM

In general, the purpose of a health care delivery system is to provide services that will maintain an **optimal health status** for the citizens of a nation, through the setting of policy and allocation of resources. The resources of the system are people, money, physical plants, and technology. The goal of a delivery system is to provide services that are accessible, appropriate, of high quality, and efficiently delivered. Many factors influence the health status of the population, such as biologic makeup, the environment in which the population resides, and life-style. In the past 10 years these factors have become more important as self-responsibility for health has become of interest to the system and to the public. However, *the design of the delivery system itself is the predominant factor that influences the ultimate state of health of the population.* The design is the driving force that influences policy decisions regarding the degree of access to care, who will receive it, how much they will receive, and who will pay for it. The design of the system is dynamic, controlled by external variables that are both political and societal. It undergoes continual scrutiny for defects that may impinge on its effectiveness. Policy changes in the system are in response to such defects and are attempts to correct them while maintaining the basic philosophy of the system. Generally these corrective responses are greatly influenced by political and economic factors, as well as by societal need and expectations.

In the United States the focal point of the design of the delivery system is expenditures for **personal health care services.** Because of this focus, the major access to the delivery system by the population traditionally has been through physician and hospital services. These two components of the system account for 67% of personal health care expenditures; long-term care accounts for 9.4%[3]; and the remainder is accounted for under the category of **other health care services.**

SYSTEM DEFECTS AS CATALYST FOR CHANGE

Health care system design is a balance between supply and demand, between resources available and resources used. Change in the system will occur as the resources for paying for health care shrink or the demands exceed the payers' ability or willingness to support the demand. Figure 1–2 demonstrates the concept of economics in health care.

When change occurs, it is often an attempt to correct some defect in the system and to adjust the balance between resources and demand for services. In the past 10 years the defect that has garnered much attention and which has had great impact on provider behavior is the prevailing method of reimbursement for health care services, **retrospective fee for service.** As the costs for providing care continued to rise despite efforts to control costs, many analysts proposed that this defect in the design of the system was the primary contributor to cost escalation. It was perceived to be a disincentive to providers to be efficient in providing services. The basic assumption of many analysts was that because the system was paying retrospectively for care based on cost to the provider for providing the service, rather than rewarding the provider for **efficiency** in providing the service, the system was contributing to the excessive cost of health care. It was suggested that if this defective method of payment were fixed by changing the method of reimbursement, greater efficiency would result and expenditures for services provided would decrease. This design defect in the system of reimbursement has become the overriding political and economic issue for the 1990s. We are currently dealing with a mixture of payment designs that combine various reimbursement approaches (e.g., fee for service, prospective payment, discounted rates). Although fee-for-service reimbursement arrangements still prevail, prospective payment philosophies and discounting approaches are gaining favor in all segments of practice. The growth of health care organizations designed for efficiency in delivery of a broad spectrum of service areas, for example, **health maintenance organizations** (HMOs) has also increased. To respond to these new concepts, the practitioner needs a clear understanding of the objectives that drive and influence the design of the system.

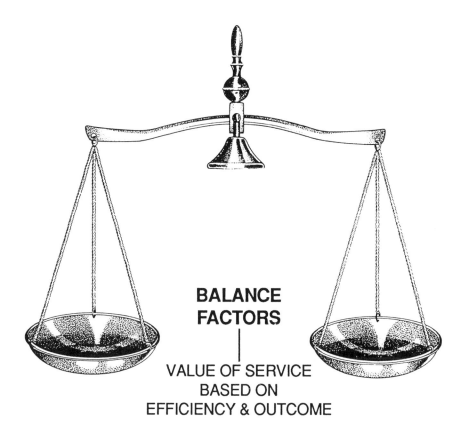

**BALANCE
FACTORS**

VALUE OF SERVICE
BASED ON
EFFICIENCY & OUTCOME

VALUE OF SERVICES
SOCIETAL DEMAND
HEALTH CARE PRIORITIES
OF THE NATION

RESOURCES AVAILABLE
GOVERNMENT
PRIVATE PAYER
BUSINESS
HOUSEHOLD (CITIZEN)

FIG 1–2.
Economics in health care is more than cost containment. The balance of demand and supply and demand, with available resources, determines which services, and to what degree, will be included or excluded. How much of societal needs will be met or what will be left unmet is determined by available resources. Inclusion or exclusion of services depends on demonstrated efficiency through outcome management.[1]

OBJECTIVES AND STRATEGIES OF A DELIVERY SYSTEM

According to one leading health care policy authority, our delivery system addresses four major objectives and strategies that influence the management of manpower, facilities, and technology[2]:

1. To supply services. This objective usually is accomplished through strategies referred to as "subsidies" (e.g., block grants; financial support as incentives for changing status).

2. To influence the demand for services to assure equitable distribution to all classes of the population through strategies such as the development of health insurance programs or entitlement (Medicare, Medicaid).

3. To alter organizations responsible for delivery of services by building new organizations to serve subgroups of the population. Examples of such strategies are the development of service organizations such as HMOs, the Veterans Administration hospital system, or rural and urban community health centers.

4. To influence the behavior of providers through regulatory control strategies.

Brown, in his paper *Health Policy in the United States: Issues and Options,*[2] suggests that today's health care delivery system design is a sum of these four objectives. The implementation of specific strategies to achieve these objectives influences the evolution of the health care system in the United States. These strategies determine how services are provided and how they are accessed by the population.

EVOLUTION OF U.S. HEALTH CARE POLICY

Brown[2] describes two major eras in the evolution of health care policy, which have brought us to the 1990s and will direct the focus of the system in the future. These are the eras of **subsidy** and **control.** We will continue to explore these concepts as they shed light on future policy agendas.

Many factors or indicators influence health care policy during any specific period of time. As the status of the indicators changes, the priorities in health care change. In addition, health care priorities are greatly influenced by the political and economic environment of the time. For example, a major indicator that has been the catalyst for change in policy recently is the federal budget deficit and rate of inflation. Today changes in health care policy are often mandated by such indicators and conditions.

1940s and 1950s—Era of Subsidy

During the 1940s and 1950s the U.S. government directed a strategy of subsidy to address three major national health priorities: to annihilate dread disease; to enhance access to services for the underserved population, especially in rural areas; and to end a perceived shortage of physicians. It is important to note that from an economic point of view, during this period the federal deficit was minimal and the rate of inflation low. The **economic indicators** supported the use of subsidies to address these priorities, because there was little concern regarding the government's financial ability to implement them. In addition, policy makers believed that to have an impact on the system, a widespread, full-scale strategy of subsidy was required if these objectives were to be met, and the resources needed would be greater than what individual states could commit.[2] One example of subsidies to increase access is the Hill Burton Grants made available for hospital construction during the 1950s and 1960s. Physician Training Capitation and Allied Health grants were also made available to address the physician shortage and to train additional workers during this period. Research grants (from the National Institutes of Health) were made available to foster research in disease and to develop technology. These subsidies seemed reasonable because the major access to health care was through hospital admissions and physician offices. To provide increased access to these resources to improve health status, more beds, more manpower, and new technology were needed. Brown[2] states that the rationale for this specific system design was that "the only thing wrong with the American health care system was that there was too little of it."

Subsidies were implemented in the 1940s and continued through the early 1970s, providing substantial monies for hospital construction and expansion, for the education of physicians and allied health professionals, and to develop technology. Although this strategy achieved the goal of increased access to health care, it also created several problems for the system, such as excessive bed capacity, especially in rural areas, and a cumbersome system operated inefficiently. Local governments and consumer groups complained that the system was not meeting their local needs because of lack of planning to assure equal distribution of and access to resources.[2] During the era of subsidy another significant factor having a pervasive influence on the problems of cost was the design for financing health care by cost-based fee-for-service. Along with this perceived defective method of reimbursement there was increased promotion and diffusion of new technology into the delivery system. With the expansion of service access through hospital construction and equipment acquisition, these costly technologies were made available to the population at large, regardless of the technology's proved efficacy or the population's ability to pay. Physicians and other health care providers had the opportunity to provide more services and to access technology through unconstrained hospital admission policies.[2] The balance between demand (volume) for services and resources available to pay for them was greatly altered as a result of subsidy.

1960s—Building Access: Payment Subsidies

In the early 1960s additional subsidies were created in response to public demand that the federal government assist citizens in paying for their health care. These **payment subsidies** were accomplished when Congress passed Social Security amendments that created the **Medicare** program for the purpose of providing assistance to the elderly and the **Medicaid** program to provide care for the poor. Along with these subsidies, special attention was given to providing access to rural populations and to special populations (e.g., children with chronic illness), again keeping in mind that these strategies were in concert with the purpose of the delivery system. The federal budget was in surplus during the 1960s, which lent support for expanded access to health care.[2] The initial financial involvement of the government in supporting health care services was negligible compared with government support in the 1990s. In 1950, national expenditures for health care constituted 4% of the **Gross National Product** (GNP). By comparison, by 1980 expenditures had risen to more than 11%, and are projected to exceed 12% of the GNP in the 1990s. The U.S. population spends approximately 14% of its income on health care, in comparison with many other countries, which spend a maximum of 10%.[4]

Raffel and Raffel[3] make the point that in addition to high expenditures, the public sector has continued to share a high percentage of total health services expenditures. This is important from the perspective that these expenditures continue to consume tax resources. Most health planners attribute federal policy directed toward building access and supportive payment subsidies as the major underlying causes of increases in government expenditures. Table 1–1 presents a graphic illustration of shift in burden of health care expenditures that has occurred as a result of health care policy designed to improve access. It also illustrates how the shift of burden to payers has occurred with change in policy directed toward cost containment.[5] Figure 1–3 illustrates dollars spent by payer category. It is interesting that 78% of the expenditures were assumed by the private sector in 1965, but by 1967 that share had dropped to 73%, with a continued decrease to 68% by 1980.[5]

According to Levit et al.,[5] this decline was due primarily to the introduction of Medicare. By 1987 the decline had reversed as the private section portion rose to 70%. A portion of this rise, according to these researchers, was attributed to the trend in 1960–1970 for increased "depth and

TABLE 1–1.

PERCENT DISTRIBUTION OF EXPENDITURES FOR HEALTH SERVICES AND SUPPLIES, BY TYPE OF PAYER: UNITED STATES, SELECTED CALENDAR YEARS 1965–1987*

Type of Payer	1965	1967	1970	1975	1980	1981	1982	1983	1984	1985	1986	1987
Total	100.0	100.0	100.0	100.0	100.0	100.0	100.0	100.0	100.0	100.0	100.0	100.0
Private	77.7	73.6	72.8	68.2	67.9	69.3	68.4	68.6	69.1	69.0	70.2	70.1
Private business	17.5	19.3	22.0	24.7	28.8	29.2	29.3	29.1	29.0	28.4	28.5	27.9
Household (individual)	58.9	53.2	49.7	42.8	38.4	39.3	38.4	38.7	39.4	39.9	41.1	41.5
Philanthrophy	1.4	1.1	1.0	0.7	0.7	0.7	0.7	0.8	0.7	0.7	0.7	0.7
Public	22.3	26.4	27.2	31.8	32.1	30.7	31.6	31.4	30.9	31.0	29.8	29.9
Federal government	10.8	14.0	14.8	17.6	17.7	16.5	17.2	17.5	17.0	17.1	16.1	16.2
State and local governments	11.4	12.4	12.4	14.2	14.4	14.2	14.4	14.0	13.9	13.9	13.7	13.7

*From Health Care Financing Administration, Office of the Actuary: Data from the Office of National Cost Estimates.

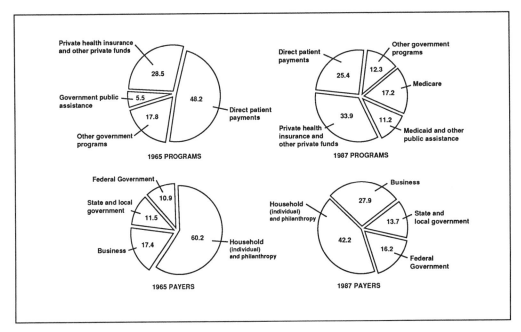

FIG 1–3.
Percent distribution of expenditures for health services and supplies, by national health accounts program and type of payer, United States, calendar years 1965 and 1987. (From Health Care Financing Administration, Office of the Actuary: *Data from the Office of National Cost Estimates.*)

breadth of employer sponsored (and largely employer paid) health insurance." This trend to offer coverage as an employee benefit is reflected in the growth in the business sector share of the burden, from 18% in 1965 to 29% by 1980. It is noteworthy that **household share**, that portion assumed by the individual, increased significantly between 1982 and 1987. Because of the excessive escalation of costs, government and business were forced to attend to decreasing their risk in supporting health care cost.[5]

1970s—Policy Changes Leading to Era of Control

During the 1970s it became clear ţhat existing health care policy had resulted in an expensive proposition that the federal government could not afford and which industry was not wholly willing to absorb. In general, it was believed that a major overhaul of the system as it related to access and cost was needed if the system were to be contained. The overriding concern was to change the provider delivery segment of the system and to modify the manner in which services were reimbursed. The preferred system in the past had been designed to pay for the cost of the service rendered in a retrospective manner, where the amount paid was based on the actual cost of providing the service. Numerous health care policy analysts continued to support and promote the principle that this method of payment was contributing to the escalation of cost. Because service costs were paid without question, there was no incentive to contain costs or to be efficient. As a result of this belief, government leaders and policy makers began to investigate ways to correct this incentive defect in the system as it applied to payment or subsidy of services. These groups favored putting in place alternatives to providing care that they believed would be less costly to sustain. The concepts of prospective pricing along with a competitive marketing were gaining favor. The intent of government was not to direct how providers deliver health care, but to find some way to reorganize the system in which they delivered the care, to control expenditures. Therefore, in essence, the 1970s became the era of **corrected incentives** to control costs.[2] The reorganization of the system to promote the agenda of efficiency resulted in the promotion of **HMOs** and **preferred provider organizations** (PPOs), **negotiated fees,** and **discounted rates.** This era led to prospective payment concepts, and more recently to selective pricing to ration care.

During this period the government began to deal with cost through government regulation by enacting legislation that created the **Health Systems Agency** (HSA) and the **Certificate of Need** process (CON). The objective of these strategies was legislative control through coordination of health planning at the local level. The intent was to ensure access to care that was appropriate and to restrict or curtail the expansion of hospitals and their acquisition of high technology equipment. These efforts, however, were met with skepticism and strong opposition, especially in the provider sector. Because of inherent weaknesses in the design of these strategies, HSAs were dissolved in the early 1980s and the CON process was deemphasized. However, some important concepts were born of these strategies, that is, *less costly alternatives of care,* and *self-responsibility for health promotion and prevention* as alternatives to a delivery system that focused on treatment of disease and illness.

In the 1970s Congress passed legislation to permit the elderly population under Medicare to join HMO organizations. This was an example of government efforts to reorganize the system to allow for access to care at less cost and in a more efficient manner. Providers initially resisted these efforts as well as efforts in the 1980s to develop PPOs and managed care concepts. Eventually most have accepted the changes in organization of service delivery and regulation within the provider community. Most providers, including physical therapists, have slowly recognized and begrudgingly accepted this shift in delivery design. Many have begun to plan and practice accordingly.

As the 1970s came to a close, the political and economic indicators in the nation began to influence policy. Subsidy during previous decades led to increased access and increased cost, and later to regulation. The system was in dire need of attention. It was clear that the cost was still affecting the ability of the system to meet its goals. The federal budget deficit and inflation continued to erode the buying power of the nation. Health care costs continued to rise regardless of efforts to reorganize the system.[2] The issues of how much of a particular health care service citizens should receive, and how and who should finance it, continued to be a matter of public debate. Likewise, providers continued to complain and resist efforts for further change. The eras of subsidy and control in the 1980s brought with them the competition aspect of health care policy. Thus began the evolution of the system known as Managed Care.[2]

1980s—Competition in the Market Place: Incentives For Efficiency Through Prospective Payment System

Federal Agenda

Brown[6] refers to the 1980s as the Decade of Transition. The federal administration ("Reaganomics") was committed to support market-based approaches to contain costs and to repeal regulatory approaches. This position was based on the belief that competition would eventually control costs as productivity and efficiency increased due to sound business practices. The hospital industry was viewed as no different from other industries; therefore, it should respond in the same manner to market strategies and approaches. According to Brown, a certain political faction, however, continued to support the strategy of "rate-setting programs" as a mechanism to control costs. Several studies indicated that this strategy was effective in containing costs.

As a result of these studies, legislation was passed that permitted and encouraged states to adopt **gatekeeping** and managed care systems to control costs in Medicare and Medicaid programs.[6] Most important, during this era (1982) Congress passed the **Tax Equity Fiscal Reform Act**, known to providers as TEFRA. This legislation was paramount in affecting health care policy. It created the prospective payment system for reimbursement to hospitals for Medicare patients and the eventual implementation of the DRG system for inpatient services. It also offered a strong dose of encouragement for reorganizing the system to make HMO development more attractive by liberalizing payments to HMOs for Medicare beneficiaries.[6] At about this time, state legislatures created statutory approval for providers and payers to form HMOs and PPOs and to negotiate fees. The concept of negotiation of contracts with selected payers was a new experience for most private practitioners. Because of the changes in reimbursement caused by these events, by the mid-1980s most physical therapists were struggling with productivity standards rather than with quality care issues. Many were faced for the first time with competing for referral sources for outpatient services. The need to change practice behavior to attend to the business aspects of patient care became an urgent reality. In terms of reimbursement, for the first time therapists were being seriously challenged regarding the efficacy of the service they provided. Payers were questioning whether the outcome achieved was of sufficient value to warrant the cost to them. Some therapists were beginning to receive denials for payment. Many expressed anger at what "The System" was doing to them. All providers have come to know the terms associated with "managed care systems." This system slowly continued to replace the traditional fee-for-service model of reimbursement. Managed care concepts have influenced the manner in which physical therapy services as well as other health care services are accessed. A major consideration for reimbursement is documented justification for the services rendered.

Private Sector Agenda

Early in the 1980s, insurance and industry became more interested in alternative systems of delivery, such as prudent purchasing and preferred provider selection. Communities began to form labor coalitions to take a more active part in addressing issues of cost containment at the local level. These groups were formed out of concern about the government's slowness in setting health policy that would control the cost escalation that had resulted from broadened access to services and increased use of technology. **Private payers** (both insurance carriers and business) had become concerned, if not alarmed, about their increased sharing of the burden or financial risk of paying for health care. This increased risk dictated financial reform in the private sector. It resulted in change in reimbursements policies and the adoption of payment incentives other than the traditional cost-based fee. Insurance policy designs began to incorporate such strategies as **co-payments, second surgical opinions, preadmission screenings,** higher **deductibles,** and **variable premium rates** based on the amount of coverage provided. With rising costs to the insurers, they in turn passed the cost of providing health care coverage to the employer in the form of increased premium rates. This cost shift, coupled with the inability of businesses, especially small ones, to pass the cost on to the consumers of their products, was the catalyst for businesses to begin looking for avenues to shift or cut costs.

As illustrated in Figure 1–3, the burden on private sector payers to support health services expenditure has increased from 18% in 1965 to 29% in 1987. According to Levit et al.,[5] in the 1980s "the watchword was a period of entrenchment." Insurance policy design reform began in earnest. New benefit designs and requiring employees to share a greater portion of insurance premiums were accepted alternatives for sharing the financial risk. At the same time, the move toward managed care (use of HMOs and PPOs), together with reliance on self-funded insurance rather than commercial carriers, began. These actions were examples of cost shift to share the financial risk, reduce utilization, and reduce the price for services.[5] This outcome was inevitable as insurance company losses were coupled with double digit inflation in the early 1980s and again in 1988. Insurance companies were forced to recoup losses by increasing premiums to employers, which drove health insurance premiums to an average $2,354 per employee per year in 1989. Small businesses were especially hard hit by these events. During the 1980s small business saw a jump in benefit costs from 20% to 150%.[7] Many employers have passed the cost on to the employee (household category of expenditures). Some have offered them **menu options** to select coverage that will meet their personal needs and to decide which services they are willing to pay for themselves. As a result of this cost shift and changes in benefit structure, many employees have elected to go without coverage. By the end of the 1980s, most sources estimated that 34% of the U.S. population (or 37 million persons) no longer had basic health care insurance coverage. During the 1990s, as the budget deficit increased and the national economy declined further, this figure has increased because of high unemployment rates. In the 1990s health care benefits continue to be a major issue at the bargaining table. They are the central focus of labor negotiation packages rather than pay raises or other benefits.

FUTURE OF HEALTH CARE POLICY

The objectives and strategies of the U.S. health care delivery system have changed significantly over the past two decades. The design of the system, however, continues to be based on access and delivery of health care services through expenditures of resources. Unless this design changes as a result of drastic health care reform, all payers, both government and private, will increase their focus on the value of the outcome for the dollars invested in health care. One way they will accomplish this is by utilizing data collected by PROs and HSAs and carriers on how health care is provided and how it is used by the consumer. From these data **practice profiles** (practice patterns related to outcome) of individual providers are being developed. These profiles are being used to make reimbursement decisions. Review of the health care environment at the end of the 1980s shows that the philosophical commitment to the delivery system, with focus on service expenditures, is intact. However, access to and quality of care for the general population have become an overriding concern of the public, labor, and industry. Before we address what lies ahead, it might be helpful to compare the old system of health care delivery, to which we have been accustomed, with the new system, in terms of philosophy, access issues, and reimbursement strategies. The major changes in focus and philosophy of these two systems are illustrated in Table 1–2.

The budget deficit of the 1980s was carried into the decade of the 1990s. It presents a consistent indicator that broad, decentralized access to health care is unaffordable under the current system design. Most health care policy analysts concur that there should be a system that incorporates the strategies of regulation and competition to curb escalation of costs. They agree that the issue of equity of access and technology must be addressed, along with greater scrutiny of value of care in terms of dollars spent. What can we look for in the future?

Our personal impressions are consistent with those of the experts, who project that two major postures will guide the system until some type of revolutionary reform occurs. These postures, regulation and mixed competition, have influenced policy over the past two decades and have created a **two-tier system** of health care delivery, with resultant multilevel access to health care. By definition, this system supports general access to a minimum standard of basic health care for citizens who cannot afford to pay for more. The minimum standard focuses on primary care and prevention. Other levels, or higher standards of care, are available to citizens who are able and willing to pay extra for them.[3, 6]

No doubt the public will continue its outcry that the system is ineffective and that total reform is needed. Some will continue to lobby that everyone should have access to all standards of care and technology regardless of ability to pay. However, at the same time the public will continue to steadfastly aver that it is unwilling to pay for such privilege through increased taxation or higher out-of-pocket expense. Politicians will profess the need for some type of universal health insurance plan. However, they will be reluctant, along with the Executive Branch of government, to impose reform, because of the presumed insurmountable financial implications for government as well as small business and industry. Individual states will attempt

TABLE 1–2.

Comparison of Systems of Health Care: 1940–1980*

Old System 1940–1970	New System 1970–1980
1. Health status outcome depends on structure and process of system design. Central focus of system is to cure illness. Improved system is equated with improved health for general population.	Nixon and Reagan administrations bring concept of HMOs, "decentralized market building," into system: a. Market competition. b. Expanded consumer choice. c. Corrective incentives provide grants to start HMOs. Goal is to "change incentives."
2. More is better; supply-side strategy; more resources: a. Biomedical research, technology, more hospitals; achieved through subsidy (NIH, Hill-Burton, legislative entitlement).	Implement centralized market building: a. Alter rules on how health insurance is bought and sold: (1) Require employers to offer choice of health plans. (2) Require equal contributions to premiums on several plans; allow employee to choose to pay for "extras" (menu options).
3. Increase access for elderly and poor through entitlement programs: a. Medicare b. Medicaid c. National health insurance (single-tier system) d. Expand system.	Question relationship of health care provision and health status outcome. Cost escalation = value for dollars expended. Life-style influences on health status: results vs spending.
4. Payment to providers based on: a. True, fair value of provider work. b. Payment based on: (1) Fee-for-service (actual cost) (2) Usual and customary fee by physicians and other providers as long as reasonable. (3) Allow medical professionals to charge what they think reasonable, within normal limits.	System too large. Unconstrained diffusion of technology leads to: a. Excessive tests. b. Excessive treatment. c. Excessive risk. d. Excessive cost. Physician glut and malpractice suits create incentive to unnecessary use and unjustified cost of care.
5. Do not implement market-based or competitive strategies to accomplish system objectives; *they do not work.*	Question desirability and affordability of entitlement programs: a. Medicare. b. Medicaid. c. *No national health insurance.* New approach through "means testing": a. Vouchers. b. Capitation. c. Higher cost sharing. d. Managed care system: (1) Multitiered system. (2) Exclude amenities. (3) Limit choice based on need and ability or willingness to pay.

TABLE 1–2 (cont.).

6. Regulation is wrong, and leads to:
   a. Inefficiency.
   b. Inequities.
   c. Perverse incentives.
   d. Sacrificed quality.
   e. Private interest control of the public.

Restructure payment system; medical decisions on use and costs are capricious.
Replace with method of objective measurement of outcome and actual cost.

7. Price competition between providers and payers will help contain costs.
   Through data systems, study use and cost patterns; identify preferred providers and prudent purchasers.
8. Regulatory controls through prospective payment to control cost of care.
   Use capital expenditure review to control technology and construction expansion.

*Adapted from Brown LD: Introduction to a decade of transition. In *Health Policy in Transition: A Decade of Health Politics, Policy and Law*. Durham, NC, 1987, Duke University Press.

to deal with the problem on a local level. Payers for health care will resist further erosion of profits by refusing to voluntarily assume responsibility for paying for more health care through employee benefit packages. They will increase efforts to reduce financial risk by passing part or all of the cost for health care coverage to their employees. In all probability, the household payer will limit insurance coverage, select plans such as HMOs to assure broader health care coverage, or go without insurance. Concepts of rationing will be entrenched throughout the system. Cost control efforts will include continued reduction in benefits in both public supported entitlement programs and by private carriers, making it more difficult for general access to all levels of care. Prospective payment and rationing methods will form the basis for reimbursement policy, especially costly high technology procedures and services, in all payer arenas. Most important, payers will insist that providers of both inpatient and outpatient services, regardless of setting, *show evidence through documentation* that the services for which they are seeking payment are effective, medically necessary, and justified. This translates as a mandate to providers to be proficient in **outcome assessment** skills. Managed care is moving toward evaluating the variation and efficacy of medical treatment outcomes to determine which produce the best results for the patient. In a recent study for *HealthWeek*, McEahern[8] investigated 25 managed care firms, and found that 52% use some degree of outcome assessment, 28% are actively exploring this method of determining appropriateness of care, 12% are currently developing such methods, and only 8% have not considered this method. She predicts that the result of research on which treatments work best will "totally shape the future of managed care."

1990s—Functional Outcome Assessment: A Measure of Health Care Value

There is little doubt that the 1990s will continue to be perceived as an era of "health care in crisis." Whatever health care reform occurs, it will continue under a managed care system design and cost containment with controlling strategies of mixed regulation and competition. The strongest indicators that will continue to greatly influence policy decisions will be the federal budget deficit, the increasing age of the population, and the debate over the philosophical issue of access to care vs who should assume the financial risk of paying for it. The divergent expectations of health care services will make reform a difficult goal to achieve because each segment of the system—provider, payer, and consumer—seems unwilling to compromise.

Recent media focus seems to indicate that reform will not come easily or quickly. While this perspective is popular currently, continued pressure by society for the government to embrace the concept of universal health coverage should not be ignored. Whatever shape reform takes in the future, it will occur. Three reform approaches, commonly referred to as the private market approach, the employee-based approach, and the government-based approach, are receiving serious consideration by business and government. All approaches promote managed care and place constraints on providers to contain costs. The major difference in the three approaches is which services will be covered and who ultimately will pay for them. With that perspective in mind, what can we as providers expect in the next decade? It might be helpful to look at some statistics that project future health care expenditures. It is likely that these projections will affect you as a provider.

Most authorities concur, somewhat cautiously, that prospective payment, market-based strategies, including competition, have had a limited positive effect on decreasing cost escalation and expenditures for inpatient hospital services and physician services. On the basis of these assumptions, it is likely that these approaches to cost containment will continue in the future. One area of noted growth that may influence future policy in the government and private payer sectors is the subcategory of "other professional services," assigned to the expenditure category of "professional services." Both of these expenditure designations are included under the general category of "personal health care expenditures." The major categories of personal health care include hospital and nursing home care, physician, dentist, and other professional services. Hospitals account for the greatest share of these expenditures, and physicians for the second largest share. Letsch et al.[9] report that although institutional spending has slowed somewhat since 1987, expenditures attributed to professional services (i.e., dentists, physicians, and other health professionals), in comparison, have shown the highest growth. However, they report that statistics show that since 1987 the category of "other professional services," which includes physical therapy services, grew faster than any other type of service. This escalation has been continuous since 1980.[9] Arnett et al.[10] report that the category of "other professional services" (freestanding home health agencies, optometrists, podiatrists, chiropractors, private duty nurses, occupational therapists, speech therapists, physical therapists, and clinical psychologists) accounted for $9 billion of expenditures in 1984, and was projected to account for $16 billion in 1990. Furthermore, this service category is expected to "experience a faster growth rate than most other personal health services."[10] Based on more recent Health Care Finance Administration data, this figure is projected to increase to $18.8 billion by the year 2000. In some instances this category of services has already become an issue of discussion. Lion et al.[11] studied the use of DRGs for hospital outpatient ambulatory surgery for Medicare beneficiaries. They propose that this system may be an appropriate strategy for cost containment in both outpatient and inpatient settings. This study was conducted in response to the recent congressional mandate that the Office of Health Care Financing Administration design a full prospective payment system for ambulatory care by 1990 and extend prospective payment system financing to all hospital-based outpatient services.[11]

Why should physical therapists be concerned about these projections? As the potential for exorcising cost savings directed at hospital inpatient services and physician offices diminishes, other professional health care services will be scrutinized for opportunities to enhance cost containment. It would be obtuse not to suggest that the category of outpatient services and professional services, in which physical therapy is included, will be ignored by either the public or the private payer sector. All providers in this category should look seriously at whether their services will stand up under such scrutiny and control.

It is tempting for physical therapists to rationalize that this system is interesting but does not really have much to do with them, inasmuch as physical therapy is such a small part of the system. Often physical therapists project an attitude that business is good and the public wants access to physical therapy services. They believe that if they concentrate only on being excellent practitioners, patients will always be there. They are convinced that if the insurance company will not pay for services the patient will. This mindset places the practice at risk. Considering the predictions of managed care for the future, it would be wise to seize the opportunity to change such attitudes and to implement practice strategies that are in concert with the delivery system. There is little doubt that rehabilitation services are valued by the public. Two questions, however, need to be addressed. First, if payers decide to ration care as a trade-off to assure "universal basic health care" to all, will payers be willing to include physical therapy as a basic service and pay for it? Second, if the government and private payers limit or will not pay for physical therapy, will the individual citizen be willing to? With the prevailing customary costs of physical therapy services and lack of evidence of efficient outcome, it is doubtful that they will.

It is certain that during the 1990s the design of the health care delivery system will be managed care and cost containment. There will be a continued focus on rationing of services to conserve resources and to achieve balance between volume and resources. The agenda will be value for the dollar invested. As a professional services provider, the profession of physical therapy is vulnerable, because too many physical therapists, despite the obvious need for system reform, still fail to use tools or skills in clinical decision making and documentation. Their documentation does not objectively measure or demonstrate that the outcome of what they do is clearly linked to appropriate and medically necessary care reflective of a medical diagnosis. Often treatment plans are not directed toward functional goals. They fail to take heed that the general orientation of policy makers and third-party payers is that managed care should focus on reducing variations in care by measuring the result of treatment. Clearly, reimbursement decisions will be made based on the value of the service provided and a demonstrated measure of the outcome achieved. The practitioner must approach patient intervention from this perspective.

Carriers do not place a high value on physical therapy services as they relate to managed care concepts. Practitioners have ignored the need to collect objective data on which to develop utilization profiles. Many physical therapists have been slow to recognize the value of clinical research. They place little importance on participating at the local level in the development of data bases to set **community standards** that can influence reimbursement policies set by payers.

Practitioners have neglected to take the lead; consequently, payers have determined reimbursement rates on their behalf. Many practitioners have been reluctant to implement quality assurance programs as well. Data collection on efficacy of treatment procedures and outcomes is pivotal in addressing the issues of value in managed care. Practitioners, for the most part, cannot demonstrate that specific physical therapy treatment regimens make a difference in the patient's functional outcome. They cannot objectively demonstrate that physical therapy intervention is more cost effective than other alternatives of care. Many therapists have yet to move from a mindset of unlimited treatment approaches to assure that the patient "gets everything he or she needs" to cure any problem to one of critically assessing problems relevant to the medical diagnosis or the patient's needs and then selecting a specific treatment regimen with functionally oriented goals that are considered medically necessary. In many instances they reject outcome assessment approaches to clinical decision making by clinging to the defense that "there are too many variables" among patients to predict the outcome of the treatment given. Efficiency is not a palatable word for many practitioners as they confuse quality of care with quantity. Inability or refusal to accept responsibility for clinical decisions that we infer will help resolve dysfunction problems is our Achilles heel. This posture sends a message that we are not confident that what we do makes a difference. This posture holds little credence in the payer arena. However, these situations are amenable to resolution.

As stated, the most rewarding aspect of being a physical therapist is to help others who are suffering from dysfunction as a result of disease or injury. This desire is a priority and the ultimate goal of every physical therapist. To achieve this goal, however, the public, payers, and other providers must be convinced that what we do is important enough and valuable enough to be included in health care services for which they are willing to pay. As so many health care analysts have postulated, all countries, regardless of the health care delivery system design, possess limited resources for the provision of health care. Based on the priorities and resources available, hard decisions must be made to balance the volume of services that can be provided against the available resources. As a practitioner, you also must work to balance the equation.

ACKNOWLEDGMENT

I thank Lawrence D. Brown, Ph.D., for permission to incorporate his views on health policy in transition in this chapter.

REFERENCES

1. Mooney G: *Economics: the road to better physiotherapy.* World Confederation of Physical Therapy, London, July 1991.
2. Brown LB: Health Policy in the United States: Issues and Options. *Bull NY Acad Med* 63:427–479, 1987.

3. Raffel MW, Raffel NK: *The United States Health System, Origins and Functions,* ed 3, Media, Pa, 1989, Harwal, p 226.

4. Wilson FA, Neurhauser D: *Health Services in the United States,* Cambridge, Mass, 1974, Ballinger.

5. Levit K, Freeland MS, Waldo DR: Health spending and ability to pay: business, individuals and government. *Health Care Financ Rev* 10:7, 1989.

6. Brown LB, editor: *Health policy in transition, a decade of health politics, policy and law,* Durham, NC, 1987, Duke University Press, Chapter 1.

7. Thomson R: Curbing costs of health care, *Nation's Business,* Sept 1989, pp 18–19.

8. McEahern S: All Eyes on Medical Outcomes, Factbook, *Healthweek,* Feb 26, 1990, p 33.

9. Letsch SW, Levit KR, Waldo DR: Health care financing trends. *Health Care Financ Rev* 10:109, 1988.

10. Arnett RH III, McKusick DR, Sonnefeld ST, et al: Projections of health care spending to 1990. *Health Care Financ Rev* 7:19, 1986.

11. Lion J, Vertrees J, Malbon A, et al: Toward a prospective payment system for ambulatory surgery. *Health Care Financ Rev* 11:79–86, 1990.

TEST YOUR KNOWLEDGE

1. Define "health care economics" and describe how this concept fits as a part of a physical therapy practice.

2. In the context of health care delivery, what two provider groups have been the primary target for cost containment in the delivery system?

3. Describe the difference between a prospective payment reimbursement system and a retrospective payment reimbursement system?

4. Name the four major policy views discussed for the future of managed care?

5. Define "managed care."

6. Name two methods used by the delivery system to control the cost of health care.

7. Describe the purpose of a health care delivery system.

8. Identify the major components of the health care delivery system in the United States, and describe the component that consumes most of its resources.

9. Name the four objectives of the delivery system discussed in this chapter, with accompanying strategies to achieve them.

10. What are the balancing factors that are the driving force for health care policy decisions?

11. What are the three major factors that have led to the excessive cost of health care over the past 40 years?

12. Explain the major dilemmas facing government, industry, and payers in providing adequate health care coverage to all aspects of the population.

13. Describe the concept of "sharing financial risk" in relation to providing for health care coverage. How has it led to the current discussion of national health care agendas?

14. What were the foci of the two major eras of evolution of health care policy that resulted in system reform during the 1980s?

15. What part did government subsidy play in causing escalation of health care costs in the United States?

16. Why are business and labor so concerned about health care costs today?

17. What does "competition in the marketplace" mean to you?

18. Describe the major policy focuses of the old system of health care delivery and the new system.

19. What is meant by a "two-tiered system" of health care?

20. Why should you be concerned about the health care system reform issues of the future?

TEST YOUR KNOWLEDGE ANSWER SHEET

1. "Health care economics" means the use of resources to ensure that society gets the best possible return in terms of human welfare from the resources available.
2. The two major groups of providers targeted for cost containment are hospitals and physicians.
3. Prospective payment reimbursement is payment based on a predetermined rate prior to provision of the service. If the provider can provide service for less than the set amount, a profit is realized. Retrospective (fee-for-service) reimbursement generally reflects the cost of providing the service as determined by the provider. It usually meets an acceptable community standard.
4. The four major policy views of managed care of the future are:
   a. Increase efforts to control cost through targeting of hospital inpatient and physician services.
   b. Increase efforts to include outpatient services as a target for cost control.
   c. Increase use of selective pricing along with modified versions of PPS as a means to ration and control access and volume of health care services.
   d. Further efforts by payers (both government and business) to share the risk of financing health care with business, labor, and households.
5. Managed care is a delivery system design that controls cost and access of health care services through a mix of regulation and competition. The focus of reimbursement is on care that is deemed medically necessary, is efficient, and is functionally related to outcome.
6. Two methods the system has used for controlling cost of health care are regulation and competition; others are selective pricing, preadmission screening, prior approval and other benefit designs, and discounted rates.
7. The purpose of a health care delivery system is to provide optimal health status to the citizens of a nation through the setting of policy and allocation of resources.
8. The major components that influence the health status of the health care delivery system in the United States are biologic makeup, environment, life-style, and design of the delivery system. The major component that consumes most of the resources is the design of the delivery system, which focuses on expenditures for personal health care services.
9. The four major objectives of the delivery system, and accompanying strategies are:

a. Subsidy, using such strategies as block grants and other means of financial support.
b. Influence demand for services, using such strategies as health insurance entitlement programs (Medicare, Medicaid).
c. Change organizations that deliver services, using such strategies as development of health maintenance organizations, VA hospitals, and rural health clinics.
d. Influence behavior of providers, using strategies such as regulatory control.

10. The balancing factor that is the driving force for health care policy decisions is value of the service, based on efficiency and outcome.

11. The three major factors that have led to excessive health care costs over the past 40 years are increased access to care, increased use of and development of technology, and method for reimbursement of payment to providers.

12. The primary dilemmas facing government, payers, and industry in their ability to provide health care coverage for the nation's citizens are:
a. Increased inflation, the federal budget deficit, and recession have eroded resources available to government to pay for subsidies and to support all aspects of the system.
b. Because of increased costs and use, payers have experienced drastic narrowing of profit margins, and have begun to pass a share of the financial risk on to business and industry.
c. Industry, especially small business, has seen an explosion in premium rates for health care. Because it can no longer pass the cost on to consumers, profit margins are shrinking. Health care has become a major expense in employee benefits packages. The employer is passing the financial risk on to the employee.

13. "Sharing financial risk" means passing the cost of covering health care services to other parties within the population, primarily government, private insurance companies, business and industry, and the household or individual. Each shares some portion of the burden to pay for services rendered.

14. The two major eras of evolution of health care policy that led to reform during the 1980s were:
a. Subsidy, which originated primarily during the 1940s and 1950s, and extended into the 1960s with the advent of entitlements that created Medicare and Medicaid. The purpose was to build access to health care services.
b. Control, which in essence was an era of corrected incentives to con-

trol costs through regulation and prospective payment approaches to reimbursement. The purpose was to encourage efficiency in provision of care.

15. The government, through subsidy programs, enhanced the construction of facilities and promoted research, which led to greater availability of technology and increased health manpower. These programs resulted in increased access to and use of services and technology by the population. The demand for and volume of services provided began to exceed the resources available.

16. Business and labor are concerned about health care costs, and health care coverage is a major issue at the bargaining table. Because of increased costs of insurance, businesses no longer can afford to absorb the high premiums and are trying to find ways to share the financial risk for providing health care coverage to employees and their families.

17. "Competition in the marketplace" refers to the premise that hospitals and other provider environments are businesses, like any other type of business. Therefore competition influences efficiency, which results in profit. Those who are most efficient will survive; others will not, because they will not be able to meet the demands (for a particular service) of the marketplace. As a result, the cost of providing the service should be lower. The more efficient the provider the less cost to provide the service.

18. The major policy focuses of the old and new systems of health care policy are:
    a. Old system, 1940–1970:
       (1) More is better; improve the system and improved care will result.
       (2) Supply-side strategies will result in better care.
       (3) To deliver care, subsidy is needed for construction, manpower, and payment (Medicare, Medicaid).
       (4) Providers are fair and should be reimbursed based on what it costs them to provide the service.
       (5) Competition is bad for the system because it compromises quality and will not accomplish system objectives.
       (6) Regulation is bad for the system because it promotes inefficiency and inequities of access. It sacrifices quality and is not in the best interest of the public.
       By 1970, as a result of cost escalation and budget deficit the focus began to shift, to begin including some forms of regulation and competition. Eventually prospective payment was put in place, along with certificate of need review.
    b. New system, 1970–1980 and beyond

(1) The decade was characterized by a decentralized market, that is, HMOs, PPOs, expanded consumer choice of coverage, and more regulation. Incentives to correct the manner in which health care services were paid for.

(2) There were altered rules for health insurance, that is, how it was paid for and sold. Employers were required to give employees a choice of plans based on what employees were willing to pay for (menu options).

(3) Entitlement programs were questioned. Were they affordable?

(4) There was implementation of means testing through higher cost sharing, capitation, and managed care. A multi-tiered system was created based on willingness and ability to pay.

(5) There was focus on restructuring of the payment system. The old system allowed physicians to make capricious decisions about cost. A method of objective measurement of value of service was implemented based on actual cost and outcome received for dollars expended.

19. In a two-tiered delivery system a basic or minimum amount of primary care is offered to all citizens. Care beyond that basic level can be accessed based on the individual's ability and willingness to pay.

20. You should be concerned about future reform issues because as a provider of rehabilitation services you are a part of the problem of cost containment and therefore must be a part of the solution. As policy decisions are made based on efficient, medically necessary care that is functionally related, you must be able to document and demonstrate that what you do is cost effective, efficient, and relevant to the expenditure of health care dollars. Along with your colleagues, you must develop use profiles that demonstrate that physical therapy services are of value to the population, are important to meeting the goals of the delivery system, and are worthy of expenditure of resources available.

CHAPTER 2

Importance of Documentation to Patient Care Reimbursement

Susan H. Abeln, P.T., A.R.M.

Key Concepts

- Know yourself and your practice
- Know the system
- Who reads our reports, and what do they want?
- Conversations about our reports and documentation
- Reimbursement considerations in reporting
- Legal considerations
- Summary

The growth of the present U.S. health care delivery system was traced in Chapter 1. That discussion illustrated the increasing number of constraints that are driving us toward a managed care system. This system has markedly increased competition among all providers for the limited dollars available for health care. And it is a system with which physical therapists appear to be at odds. Some indeed are struggling to survive.

Several quotations from a Chinese philosopher, Sun Tzu, written over 2500 years ago, seem pertinent. His now classic words are found in a work titled *The Art of War*.[1] This treatise, now widely accepted as a guide to successful leadership, offers insight into struggles, especially those for survival. They are:

- "The true object of war is *peace*."
- "Supreme excellence consists in breaking your enemy's resistance without fighting."
- "He will win who knows when to fight and when not to fight."
- "If you know neither the enemy nor yourself, you will succumb in every battle."
- "If you know yourself but not your enemy for every victory gained you will also suffer a defeat."
- "If you know the enemy and know yourself, you need not fear the result of a hundred battles."

We realize we are not at war with the U.S. health care system; however, words about war can be applied to struggles such as ours. Because the system and the **third-party payers** control the cash we must have to pay staff, purchase new equipment, lease space, and make a living by practicing our profession, survival requires us to work effectively and efficiently within the constraints of the system. Therefore, like Sun Tzu, we propose that we physical therapists look more closely at ourselves and our practices as well as at the system, **managed care,** and third-party payers so that we do not find ourselves racing blindly into a situation many have equated to a battlefield.

KNOW YOURSELF AND YOUR PRACTICE

Philosophers and psychologists for years have discussed different methods for truly knowing oneself. They frequently resort to asking a number of questions. The answers to these questions are then analyzed and discussed. This process is often interesting and enlightening. Therefore we ask you to think about your answers to the following questions and listen to your mental responses. Our reason for doing this is to provide you some insight into your physical therapy practice.

- Are you a good physical therapist?
- Do you provide "quality" care?
- What is quality in the context of physical therapy?
- Does quality care mean:
    Care provided by a clinician who has participated routinely in professional development experiences?
    Care that generates therapist or staff satisfaction?
    Care that is provided by the same therapist or practitioner?

      Care that meets the standard of care in my community/region or nationally?
- What would this type of "quality" look like in your practice?
- Do you believe this kind of care is demonstrated in your practice?
- Does the presence of your concept of "quality" guarantee that your patients are satisfied with your treatment or the care you have provided them?
- Would your patients come to you again?
- What do your patients think of you?
- What do your patients think is good, or "quality," care and service? (Have you asked them?)
- Do they think good (quality) care and service is
  Care that adds to the general well-being of the patient?
  Care that provides symptomatic relief to the patient?
  Care that meets or exceeds patient expectations for the treatment?
  Care that generates patient satisfaction?
  Care that meets key customer satisfaction issues for the patient?
- Do you believe this type of care is demonstrated in your practice?
- Do your patients "get well"?
- Does their physical functioning improve?
- Does that mean good (quality) care and service is:
  Care that effects complete resolution of the objective findings?
  Care that leads to improved clinical outcome?
  Care that leads to a quantifiable functional improvement?
  Care that generally improves the health status of the patient?
- Do you believe this type of care is demonstrated in your practice?
- Do your patients believe this type of care is being given?
- How much of the revenue of your practice, or your income, comes from your patients?
- How much revenue comes from other payer sources?
- Who are these other payers?
- What do these sources think of you?
- How do they form their opinions about you?
- Do they think that good/quality care and service is:
  Care that is appropriately and completely documented?
  Care that leads to quantifiable functional improvement within the limits of reimbursement?
  Care that lowers the total work days lost due to an injury or illness?
  Care that makes the maximum possible contribution to the reduction of lost productivity?
  Care that is cost-efficient?

- Do you believe this type of care is demonstrated in your practice?
- Do the patients believe this?
- Do the other payer sources believe this?
- Do they think your practice gives good (quality) care?
- Are they satisfied with your treatment or care of the patient?
- Do they think you get your patients well?
- Are you sure?

Others' Perspectives on Physical Therapy

Only you can answer the questions we have posed. Unfortunately, others are also asking and answering these questions. As physical therapists who routinely work with insurance claims representatives and utilization review nurses, we have been aghast at the comments these persons make when asked about physical therapy services and physical therapists. For example:

- Do they ever get anyone well?
- Why do they need to do five things for each treatment?
- They usually have poor documentation of goals and progress, and there is poor objective data.
- They seem to base a lot on complaints of pain.
- They treat until death do us part.
- Physical therapists are the worst abusers in the health care system.

What causes these people to have such strong negative feelings about our profession? Do they have or have they had any formal training about physical therapy prior to making such judgments? Usually not. The opinions and the payment decisions they make are based on the billings, documentation, and reports they routinely see from physical therapists.

Need to Modify

Documentation and reporting have always been viewed as something physical therapists just have to do. So we do it. Some physical therapists write copious, overly detailed reports on routine events; some write in technical jargon or PT-ese; others write notes so spartan that full sentences are as scarce as hen's teeth. In the past we have not written—and even now do not write—reports for those outside our profession. Yet it is these people who control our destiny. The strong negative reactions to our reports cited previously provide a clear signal that *now is the time to change and/or modify our approach to documentation*. We can no longer afford to "just do it."

All physical therapists need to know and understand who reads our reports, why they think the way they do, and what they want. We need to improve our documentation and reporting skills to "break their resistance without fighting."

KNOW THE SYSTEM

Value Equals Quality Divided by Cost

Each day the newspapers and magazines remind us of the rapid increase in health care costs and their effects on such things as union negotiations, profit lines of major businesses, and workers' compensation costs. Further, the media have begun to proclaim the need to increase the value of health care and are echoing the battle cry of many **purchasers** for new ways to reduce costs.

According to *Business & Health* magazine, "Purchasers of health care know they need to improve the value of what they are buying from the health care marketplace. They have been trying to do that for years. In the 1980s, the cost side of the equation $V = Q \div C$ (value equals quality divided by cost) was attacked with vigor, primarily through discounting."[2]

Discounting, however, resulted only in cost shifting and had very little if any effect on inflation of health care costs. Only since 1988 has the purchaser of health care begun to use the other part of the equation—the definition and measurement of quality—using **outcomes management** as a method to improve the value of what they were purchasing.

Outcomes Management

Outcomes management is a fairly new term, and definitions vary. According to Taulbee,[2] "Generally it involves gathering and analyzing the results of medical processes and performances and then using that data to manage health care provision." These data come basically from providers' billings, medical documentation, and reporting. The premise that the system must change in order to reward efficiency and effectiveness is based principally on this same information. This concept of outcome management was introduced by Ellwood, and has become a valuable management tool. This method has allowed employers and payers to "work together with providers to purchase health care more effectively and ultimately to purchase more effective health care. With the information gained, the goal (of the purchasers ultimately) is to change the incentives in the health care system to reward efficiency and effectiveness."[2]

According to one medical expert, the result of the movement to an outcome management system is that purchasers and many cost-conscious providers are looking for treatment programs designed and based on "outcomes that are known to aid patients in returning to normal function, both medically and socially in the shortest period of time."[3]

Such programs should be based on "guidelines synthesized from the medical literature, both biologic and sociological in order to determine the most efficient manner of making a specific diagnosis, which in turn can lead to a detailed therapeutic program. Such a program is not only patient-conscious, but cost-conscious, leading to a win-win-win situation for the patient, payer, and society."[3]

As physical therapists we support win-win situations. Because documentation and reporting form the base that drives the outcomes management process, we must strive to improve documentation. Our reports must clearly articulate to payers that physical therapy services are effective and efficient and that the outcome is worth the dollar spent. *One important aspect of understanding the system and achieving successful reimbursement is understanding who reads our reports and what these readers want.* Now we will turn our attention to third party payers, purchasers, managed care companies and others outside our profession, such as attorneys, who have an impact on our lives. This chapter will examine commonalities between all third party payers as the move to managed care continues.

WHO READS OUR REPORTS, AND WHAT DO THEY WANT?

Your documentation and reports, whether sparse and sloppy or detailed, objective, and complete, will cross many desks (Table 2–1). What you write and how you write it will influence others' opinions about your capability and the capability of the profession to provide effective and efficient health care. It also may cause others to generalize about the entire practice of physical therapy, as seen in the comments of the insurance claims representatives and utilization review nurses already quoted. It is important to keep in mind most of the individuals named in Table 2–1 have never and probably will never have any formalized training or inservices to assist them in understanding what physical therapy is, what constitutes physical therapy expertise, how effective we are, what areas we evaluate, what different treatment approaches we utilize, the extent of our education, how autonomously we practice, what means we use to develop and monitor our treatment plans, and how efficient we are in obtaining patient recovery or return to function with different diagnoses.

TABLE 2–1.

SOME READERS OF PHYSICAL THERAPIST NOTES AND REPORTS

Primary and referring physicians	Group Health claims representatives
Physician's nursing staff	Group Health claims auditors
Other physical therapists	Medical bill review service staff
Occupational therapists	Auditing firms
JCAHO representatives	Malpractice defense attorneys
CARF representatives	Malpractice defense attorney's staff
Utilization review nurses	Malpractice plaintiff attorneys
Utilization review physicians	Malpractice plaintiff attorney's staff
Technicians involved in claims review	Jury members
Preferred provider organization staff	Judges
Physical therapy peer review companies	Expert witnesses for the defense
State examining committee staff	Expert witnesses for the plaintiff
Fraud investigators	Potential expert witnesses for either side
Social services staff	HMO staff
Discharge planners	Medicare intermediary review nurses
Home health agencies	Medicare intermediary review therapists
Workers' Compensation technicians	Preferred provider organization utilization
Workers' Compensation claims adjusters	Review
Workers' Compensation supervisors	Physical therapy preferred providers
Workers' Compensation auditors	Utilization review team members

JCAHO = Joint Commission on Accreditation of Hospitals, CARF = Commission on Accreditation of Rehabilitation Facilities, HMO = health maintenance organization.

Most **readers** of our reports have taken a course or two on general medical terminology, but probably have never had any detailed instruction in anatomy or how or why a quadriceps-hamstring torque ratio justifies the "need" for continued therapy. Consider an attorney who has spent 4 to 6 years becoming educated in the labyrinthine processes of law; despite this, he or she would certainly not have a detailed understanding of how a muscle grade of P− for the anterior tibialis means anything to the patient's ability to resume major life activities.

Consider a note (Fig 2–1) sent to Linda, a claims examiner working in a preferred provider organization (PPO) to explain the "need" for continued therapy after 6 months and countless dollars expended. The physical therapist *assumed* that she understood a great deal about physical therapy. Linda, a high school graduate with *one* 2-hour medical terminology class and 6 months working experience, had no understanding of anatomy or pathology. She alone holds the purse strings for payment of therapy bills. It is not surprising that because she could make no sense of this note, further therapy was denied and all payments for the past 2 months of treatment that had been held pending this report also were denied! If it is true that "the meaning of any communication is defined by the response it elicits,"[4] this effort to communicate "need" for further therapy to an insurance represen-

To Whom It May Concern:

Mr. A. has been receiving physical therapy since August 22, 1988, for diagnosis sympathetic reflex dystrophy following lumbar sympathectomy. Treatment has focused on increasing strength and mobility of left lower extremity, particularly quadriceps, gluteals, and gastrocnemius. He is making slow but steady progress. Mr. A. would benefit from continuation of physical therapy program. Goals of treatment are to increase quadriceps strength to G+; increase gastrocnemius and anterior tibial musculature strength to G+; increase endurance to ambulation and activity such that Mr. A. could maintain a 4-hour activity level.

In my professional opinion, physical therapy should be continued on a monthly basis, with monthly reassessments to be made with regard to his continuation.

P.T.

FIG 2–1.
This note to a claims examiner is too general to convey the patient's status and physical therapy requirements.

tative failed miserably. And if this representative was asked her comments on physical therapists, don't you think her comments would echo those listed earlier?

Does this note communicate the following to you, as a health care provider?

- How much progress this patient had made
- Over what course of time
- What his muscle scores were at the time the letter was written
- What these scores had to do with the patient's ability to function in his life
- How much longer the therapist expects treatment to be continued

All we can tell from this report is that the patient is supposed to be slowly progressing. It is difficult to ascertain whether the patient could stand when he began treatment, or can stand now. Could he ambulate at all when treatment began? Is he ambulating now? Over what distance? If he is ambulating, is he using any assistive device? It is not easy to tell how an increase in strength of the patient's quadriceps and anterior tibialis strength to G+ will influence his function. In general, all we know is where this patient's treatment is headed. The things we don't know include where treatment of the patient's condition began, where it is now, how long a trip it will be, or what the final destination is.

The resultant feeling of frustration and confusion can be likened to a travel agent's being told only that his or her client wanted to continue a trip to Los Angeles, without being told:

- Where the trip began (e.g., New York City, Miami, Chicago, or Santa Barbara?)
- Where the client is now (e.g., Philadelphia, New Orleans, Denver, or Hollywood?)
- How long he wanted this trip to take (should it be on motor scooter, bus, train, or plane?)
- How much money he expected to spend

The note shown in Figure 2–2, dated June 10, was sent to an employer who, in accordance with his state law, was funding all payments for work-related injuries from regular operation accounts. In other words, this employer had *no* Workers' Compensation insurance coverage and had chosen to pay for any lost wages *and* any injured employee's bills *he thought appropriate* out of his monthly cash flow. This employer had only one significant injury to an employee within the past year, a back injury to a 5' 1", 205-lb woman named Laura B. Gene, the individual who has the responsibility to make the determinations on payments to providers (one reader of this note), is a human resource specialist for the employer. Gene has a masters degree in Business Administration, and minimal medical knowledge. When he realized that the current drain on his employer's cash flow from Laura's case was significant, Gene asked for a report from the physical therapist providing treatment. He needed to get some sense of the employee's problems and what was being done to remedy those problems. He had to know how much longer any treatment would take and how much money the employer would have to fund out of his budget in a tight financial year. The employer has made available for Laura a modified work assignment that will allow for variable work position and no lifting, carrying, pushing, or pulling. When can she be expected to return to work?

On your review of this note, can you answer Gene's questions? Could Gene know how much longer Laura's treatment will continue? Could he estimate (with his background) whether the employee would be able to return to the workplace? Could he understand which treatment was being directed toward improving this employee's gait and ability to stand, and what edema in the sacral area has to do with Laura's function, her job, and her life?

These notes may not reflect your current style of reporting, but believe us they are real (the names have been changed)! These examples demon-

Laura B. has been seen as an outpatient from _____ to present. Patient injured her lower back on 10/26 while transferring a patient from bed to chair. Initial evaluation: inability to stand erect. Patient's trunk was in a forward flexed position with her knees slightly bent. Patient also had upper back symptoms initially.

- Pain: Palpation to lumbosacral area
- Gait: Decreased stance phase on right and shortened step length on left
- Edema: Sacral region
- Sensation: Tingling sensation radiating down the right leg; shooting pains in right leg with ambulation
- Range of motion: Trunk flexion, with rotation and sidebending, limited by 75%. Patient is unable to do trunk extension
- Strength: Not evaluated at this time due to the patient's pain level.

Initial physical therapy included ultrasound, electric stimulation, ice, posture and body mechanics instructions, prone on elbows, and gluteal isometrics. Patient was instructed in a home TENS unit, which she continues to use on a daily basis. Patient has been given a written exercise program. Other modalities used included iontophoresis and initiation of other trunk and lower extremity exercises. These exercises increased her low back pain.

Currently, Ms. B. exhibits difficulty with sit to stand transfers and inability to bear weight pain free evenly on her feet. She demonstrates no ilium movement bilaterally with the step test, and has pain on palpation at both the PSIS and ASIS areas. In addition, she has a 2.2-cm leg length discrepancy (right greater than left). This possibly indicates a bilateral sacroiliac dysfunction.

Treatment at this time includes ultrasound, gentle sacroiliac joint mobilization with the patient sidelying, ice, gluteal isometrics, hip extension, and knee flexion strengthening exercises prone and standing. This patient continues to use the TENS unit. She has made improvements with gait, transfers, posture, decreased edema in the lumbosacral area, and decrease in the amount of pain of lumbosacral soft tissue to palpation. She is making slow progress with the exercise routine. She currently wears a Velcro belt for SI joint support.

It appears that Ms. B. is having a difficult time with her injury. If you have any questions, please contact me at 555-1212.

FIG 2–2.
This note to an employer, although more detailed than that in Figure 2–1, fails to convey information from the viewpoint of the employer regarding the employee's current and projected functional status and prognosis for return to work, and does not offer the employer insight into the rationale of past, current, or future therapy.

strate that the challenge for physical therapists is to communicate in such a way that they demonstrate to payers their unique body of knowledge, training, and abilities to provide effective and efficient care. The strongest tool each of us has at our disposal is our documentation. As stated earlier, to many readers, your reports represent you. They will seriously influence your practice, your future practice, and our profession. Now the question remains: What do purchasers and the other readers insist on seeing in our reports and documentation?

CONVERSATIONS ABOUT OUR REPORTS AND DOCUMENTATION

We would like to share with you some key points from conversations each of us has had with purchasers in the last year:

A top level executive with a *Fortune 500* restaurant company, who is nationally responsible for selecting providers to treat injured employees and assist in development of the company's PPO network for medical coverage, explained that his company looks for providers who are available during the company's hours of business and who provide quality care. His definition of quality is based on how well and how often the therapist communicated and reported to the company and to the company's insurance carrier regarding the functional improvement of his employee. A key representative from his insurance program explained that her team determines which physical therapists get the business based on how goal oriented and goal driven the care is from a vocational or functional standpoint as well as how regularly the therapist reports this information to them in a form they can understand.

· · ·

A Risk Manager for a Fortune 500 self-insured health care company, who is responsible for the national selection of providers to treat employees with work injuries, expanded on what the ideal reports from providers including physical therapists would entail when she stated:

I would expect legible writing (typing would be great) and standardized abbreviations and symbols. With the first bill I receive I would expect:
- The complete history taken by the caregiver
- A clear statement of the problem (in terms I can understand)
- A plan of action that addresses that problem
- The expected result of that plan (function means more to me than other things) and how long the plan is going to take to achieve that result.

She had several other comments that may also be of interest:
- If they send me a bill and want me to pay it, I need to know *why?*
- They have to address the areas I want to know about!
- We choose doctors and providers by the way they report to us and the language they use.

Many states allow an employer or insurer to direct an injured worker to specific medical providers. A Workers' Compensation claims reviewer, who enforces this rule of direction, routinely judges providers by their reports to her. The following is an excerpt of one of her letters to a provider, which details an ideal report:

> In your report, I request that the following information be included:
>
> 1. What is the patient's current condition?
> 2. Is the patient currently disabled? If so, please state if the disability is temporary or permanent.
> 3. If the patient is capable of performing some type of work, please outline the restrictions that the patient presently has.
> 4. At what point in time might the patient reach a maximum level of improvement?
> 5. Please discuss the nature and extent of the patient's current medical care and probable length of time that this care will continue.

Another explanation of an ideal report was given by a utilization review nurse responsible for the review and acceptance or denial of all **flagged** medical PPO claims for a company-based PPO with more than 70,000 lives.

> What I would like to see initially is
>
> - A clear statement of what the problem is in terms I can understand
> - What you are going to do about it
> - How much time will it take you to achieve that
> - How often you will evaluate to see if what you are doing is working

She further explains:

> After the first 2 weeks, I want to know what is going on and the progress you have made
>
> Every month (at least) I would like to know the problem, the progress you have made, and what are you going to do about the remaining problem(s)
>
> At 3 months I would like to know what is taking you so long!

Another utilization review nurse who works with **Independent Physician Associations** (IPAs) and often serves as a consultant to develop cost containment and **utilization review criteria** and programs for major self-insured employers throughout the country stated the same thing in a slightly different way. He explained that "the reviewer's goal is to see that only those dollars are expended that need to be. . . Basically I want to know *what* you are doing, *why* you are doing it, and for *how much longer* you will be continuing." He also mentioned that the explanation the therapist provides must be in terms easily understood and that **discrete measurements** must be translated to something he can tell has meaning in a patient's life, such as functional abilities. Perhaps Susan Griffith, Director of Rehabilitation for Pennsylvania National Insurance Groups, distilled these comments during her presentation to the Private Practice Section's November 1990 Conference when she stated, "The one thing your profession is judged on is **outcome.**"

The preceding paragraphs have described in basic terms what both employers, as nongovernment purchasers, and third-party payers believe should be components of any report. We agree. We will look more specifically at Medicare's requirements as they relate to functionality and reporting in Chapter 5.

In summary, the ideal initial report, from the payer's perspective, includes:

- A clear statement of the problem(s), in terms understood by all readers, and discussion of the effect on function
- A plan of action that directly addresses the problem(s)
- The expected result in terms of function, and including how long the treatment will take

The ideal interim report includes:

- Restatement of the initial problem
- What you have done
- Why you have done it
- How what you have done has been effective in changing the initial problem and function
- How much longer you will have to treat the patient

REIMBURSEMENT CONSIDERATIONS IN REPORTING

When in physical therapy school, most of us were taught to view documentation of patient care as a way to communicate to other health care practitioners our diagnosis and course of treatment and to establish coordination and continuity of care. In this context reports must accomplish the following:

1. Provide documentation of patient assessments and assistance in planning patient care
2. Evaluate the patient's current condition and specify ongoing treatment
3. Allow assessment of developing patterns in patient condition
4. Provide a medical history for future admissions.

This approach to documentation and reporting is no longer enough. In addition to these basic elements, the managed care delivery system and its emphasis on outcomes requires other considerations in our reporting such as:

- Translating complex professional concepts into a form and language that can be understood easily by others outside the profession.
- Clearly stating the problem or diagnosis in readily understandable terms.
- Basing the treatment on resolving the problem identified and moving the patient to a specific functional result.
- Providing a timeline for achieving that functional outcome or result through the treatment plan. If the plan is not effective in moving the patient toward that goal, frequent re-evaluation and modification of the initial plan are expected.
- Clearly demonstrating the therapist's unique capability when dealing with each specific problem or diagnosis and demonstrating the efficacy of our treatment approach.
- Recognizing that medical records are widely used as business records and sources of information by insurance companies as well as utilization review/management firms.

These six points are discussed in the following sections.

Translating Complex Professional Concepts Into Form and Language Understood Easily by Those Outside the Profession

A recurring theme in the earlier comments from purchasers is the need for physical therapists to *translate* their thoughts and findings in lay terms. Too often, reports are written in PT-ese or even in the jargon of each speciality. Readers outside the profession can make no sense of the patient's problem or the current choice and progression of treatment. This predicament brings to mind a question posed recently by a colleague. She asked, "What good does it do to make great clinical decisions, if you are unable to communicate that ability to the community? And further, what good is a beautiful report or beautiful documentation if it does not show relevance of the evaluation and treatment to the medical diagnosis?" This section focuses on the first of these questions.

As physical therapists we begin our patient interactions with a detailed decision-making process related to that patient's condition. This process is grounded in the art and science of physical therapy. The steps in this decision making usually are documented in the scientifically based terminology we have learned so well. We can no longer assume that those outside our profession understand the nuances or combination of signs and symptoms that lead us from evaluation to assessment of the patient's functional limitations, to differential physical therapy assessment or diagnoses, and to a treatment plan. We need to make all of our documentation readily *translate* the physical findings (e.g., such as muscle scores, quadriceps-hamstring torque ratios, right/left shifts) into **functional limitations** (e.g., inability to ambulate, pain limiting ability to perform job duties). Then we must develop a treatment plan that addresses these functional limitations.

To provide a better understanding of what we mean by "translating" findings through an assessment process to functional limitations, then "translating" functional limitations to treatment, let's look at a few examples:

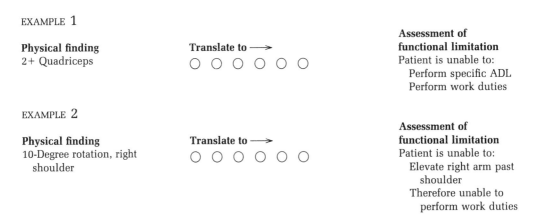

EXAMPLE 1

Physical finding   **Translate to** ⟶   **Assessment of functional limitation**
2+ Quadriceps

Patient is unable to:
   Perform specific ADL
   Perform work duties

EXAMPLE 2

Physical finding   **Translate to** ⟶   **Assessment of functional limitation**
10-Degree rotation, right
  shoulder

Patient is unable to:
   Elevate right arm past
    shoulder
   Therefore unable to
    perform work duties

The final step in this translation is to move beyond the patient's functional limitation to the treatment plan. This last translation completes the demonstration of clinical decision making and shows how the treatment approach you have decided on is based on the limitation in the patient's function. Continuing with the examples above:

EXAMPLE 3
**Assessment of
functional limitations**   **Translate to** —→   **Treatment**
Patient is unable to: ○ ○ ○ ○ ○ ○   Needs home exercise program that
  Perform specific ADL   includes_____
  Perform work duties   Needs additional assistance with ____
                                                             Needs modified work, e.g., _____

EXAMPLE 4
**Assessment of
functional limitations**   **Translate to** —→   **Treatment**
Patient is unable to: ○ ○ ○ ○ ○ ○   Needs home exercise program that
  Elevate right arm past   includes_____
    shoulder   Needs shoulder mobilization, e.g., ___
  Therefore unable to perform
    work duties   Needs modified work, e.g., _____

Such translation should allow all those who read our notes, regardless of their background, to understand our assessment of the patient's condition, how we are going to treat it, and the end result we expect to achieve, and over what course of time, as a result of our intervention. Follow one more example from clinical finding through assessment of functional limitation to treatment:

EXAMPLE 5

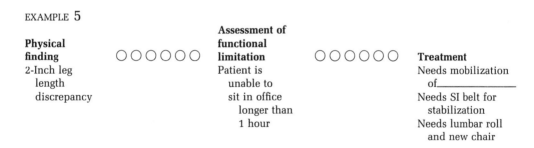

**Physical
finding**   **Assessment of
funtional
limitation**   **Treatment**
2-Inch leg   ○○○○○○   Patient is   ○○○○○○   Needs mobilization
  length   unable to   of_____
  discrepancy   sit in office   Needs SI belt for
                     longer than   stabilization
                     1 hour   Needs lumbar roll
                                                         and new chair

Chapter 3 examines in depth one particular system and the use of this clinical decision-making model to translate complex issues into a treatment program that is easily understood. Chapter 4 discusses the need to translate and review different systems that have been developed to move one step beyond current reporting using a clinical decision-making model.

Clearly Stating Problem or Diagnosis in Readily Understandable Terms

As physical therapists, each of us has been in the position of trying to make someone else (usually a physician) believe that a particular treatment intervention or identification of a critical problem was their own idea. Consequently, we each left the interpretation of our findings out of our reports. Each report was filled with enough objective data to point the way to the conclusion, so we could be certain that any reader could and would come to the same conclusion regarding a problem list or diagnosis that we, as physical therapists, had made. This tactic has often been disappointing. One instance can illustrate this. We had a conversation with "Annie," a Workers' Compensation claims adjuster who was 25 years old. She had begun her work in Workers' Compensation insurance at the age of 18 as a mail room clerk, and had worked her way up to a claims adjuster. She was certified in her state as an adjuster and could and did write checks for payment of any bill, medical or other, up to $25,000 without approval. One day after hearing her comments about a physical therapist's intervention with one of her claimants we asked her, out of curiosity, to interpret a report recently submitted to us for claims review. This report, like ours of long ago, pointed to a conclusion but did not state it. The report concerned a patient who had sudden onset of pain and "electricity" radiating down his left leg after he twisted his back while trying to mount a television as part of his regular duties at the cable company. The report went on to describe his physical findings as muscle grades of "poor minus" (2−) for both the extensor and flexor hallucis longus muscles on the left, normal muscle grades on the right, corresponding changes in sensation both to light touch and pinprick on the left, and decreased left ankle jerk reflex. In addition, the report detailed the patient's severe spasm and muscle guarding in the paravertebrals from L2 to the coccyx. There was no mention of functional limitations. Annie's conclusion, after reading these extensive, detailed, objective findings that pointed *clearly* to a specific but *unstated conclusion*, was shocking. Unlike the physical therapy interpretation, her interpretation of this report was that this gentleman, who was nearing retirement, was a malingerer who had no functional limitations and therefore could return to his full duties immediately. Her recommendation, had he been one of her claimants, would have been to deny his injury and cut off his medical benefits *and* his lost time benefits. This experience demonstrates that years of clinical practice must be rethought. It is clear from this episode that physical therapists need to include as a final part of the evaluation process a definite and clear statement of the assessment of the problems and/or physical therapy diagnosis. Further, we need to discuss the functional limitations that result from a diagnosis. We can no longer leave anything to inference.

Basing Treatment on Resolving the Problem Identified and Moving to a Specific Functional Result

Earlier in this chapter, we shared excerpts from conversations with a variety of payers. Each time one of these individuals described the ideal report they proposed **linear progression** from problem to treatment. The preceding section on translation further reinforces this need to tie the treatment to the identified problem or problems. This would seem to be a common practice, yet in chart reviews and peer reviews we have not found it to be so. Let us examine a few notes and then make modifications to demonstrate simple techniques that can be used to assure that a linear step from problem to treatment is a common practice in reporting.

The note to an insurance carrier is shown in Figure 2–3. The carrier had no knowledge of which extremity was involved, nor what the muscle scores meant overall, let alone what the scores meant in terms of this patient's functional level. Further, the treatment approach—especially the swimming, BAPS board, Theraband, and balance board—did not follow logically from these incomprehensible scores. Modifications are suggested in Figure 2–4. These modifications in language translate the complex manual muscle test results into easily understood problems. They show that the treatments recommended in the treatment regimen are logical and are designed to resolve the patient's functional limitations.

Providing a Timeline for Achieving Functional Outcome or Result Through Treatment Plan

It is probably safe to assume that at some point in our lives all of us have had bills to pay and that we did not have an infinite amount of money with

---

On manual muscle testing, the peronei are graded at 3–/5, anterior tibialis and toe extensors 1+/5, gastroc-soleus at 4–/5, posterior tibialis at 3+/5. Hip abductors are slightly weaker on MMT to that of opposite side, and he still displays a gluteus medius limp, particularly with fatigue. Patient is progressing with his Theraband exercise program and walking and swim program. Treatment will now add BAPS Board activities and balance board training.

A. Doing well

P. To continue

M Feelgood, PT

FIG 2–3.
Clinical summary report to a physician and the patient's employer does not demonstrate physical therapy rationale for extended care and apparent extensive use of passive or paliative therapy.

On manual muscle testing of right lower extremity, the peronei muscles are graded at 3−/5, anterior tibialis and toe extensors 1+/5, gastroc-soleus at 4−/5, posterior tibialis at 3+/5. Patient has improved in his control of foot drop, which is now apparent only after ambulating greater than 100 ft. But ankle lateral instability continues, so he is unable to ambulate more than 25 ft without reinjury. This is complicated by the patient's right hip abductor muscles, which are weaker on MMT to that of opposite side (2+ on R vs 4− on L). The patient still displays a gluteus medius limp, particularly with fatigue, which increases ankle instability and chance of reinjury. This has led to patient's inability to ambulate outside the house without crutches. Current treatment is focused on increasing ankle and hip strength and endurance while limiting opportunity for reinjury. Further emphasis is placed on coordination and proprioceptive retraining. Patient's BAPS Board activities, Theraband exercise program, and walking and swimming programs focus on increasing ankle and hip strength and endurance while limiting opportunity for reinjury. Balance board training, "sprain" board activities, and BAPS Board address coordination and proprioceptive retraining.

A. Patient is doing well. He has progressed in distance of safe ambulation from 10 ft to 25 ft.

P. To continue progressive exercise program for 5 more weeks at a frequency of four therapy sessions per week for the first 2 weeks, decreasing to two sessions per week after that, with extensive home pool and gym use. Anticipate patient's return to preinjury safe ambulation of 300 ft and safe stair climbing within that time.

M Feelgood, PT

FIG 2−4.
This clinical summary allows the reader to see that the treatment provided was designed to resolve objectively identified problems and move toward a specific functional result.

which to pay them. So we were forced to make choices. These choices included what to purchase, how to pay for it, to pay for it now or over time, over what period of time to pay for the product or service, and when to stop paying because the value of the product or service was less than the price paid. The last two questions are the ones that are haunting when shopping for a car. How long will that car payment need to keep being paid? Is there a point when the value of that car is less than the remaining payments? This situation is very much like the one claims adjusters or utilization review nurses have faced in reviewing claims for the past 10 years. The questions of how long they must go on paying for a service and has the product or service reached a point of diminishing value are also troublesome issues for them. In other words, like us, they have been forced to make choices. They can make better choices if we provide them with critical information to assist in addressing these nettlesome questions. What are they asking for? Simply stated, most purchasers want to know the expected functional result of your intervention and how long the treatment is going to take to achieve that result. They realize that each patient is an individual. They also realize that physical therapy, indeed medicine itself, is not an exact science. However, physical therapy is based on science, and science is predictable. It is possible to say that most low back pain sufferers will recover with or without intervention in 6 weeks; isn't it also possible to provide a general timeline for other conditions? In your initial evaluation, you should provide a predicted timeline for treatment needed to achieve the functional outcome. This estimate should also help to monitor the effectiveness of the treatment intervention and modify the therapeutic regimen in a timely manner to effect the best result for the patient. Of course, this timeline can be modified as needed in interim reports. But keep in mind: all timeline modifications should have a rationale within the same document to explain the change. As timelines are modified, corresponding alterations in functional outcome should be reexamined. Throughout this process, it is important to remember one of the fundamental rules of customer service: underpromise and overdeliver.

Clearly Demonstrating Therapist's Unique Capability When Dealing With Each Specific Problem or Diagnosis and Demonstrating Efficacy of Treatment Approach

Physical therapists have a unique education and therefore unique capabilities. We are educated as the experts in the neuromuscular skeletal system. Our education is rigorous, and by the end of our academic course work we are well prepared to practice the art and science of physical therapy. The Board of Directors of the American Physical Therapy Association (APTA) has published a model definition of physical therapy that details the components of the art and science of this specialization. This definition emphasizes the clinician's ability to identify, detect, assess, prevent, correct, alleviate, and limit physical disability, movement dysfunction, bodily malfunction, and pain from injury, disease, and any other bodily and mental conditions. The statement also includes the provision of consultative, educational, and other advisory services for the purpose of reducing the incidence and severity of physical disability, movement dysfunction, bodily malfunction, and pain.[5] This definition portrays the art and science of physical therapy practice, inclusive of documentation.

The problem or challenge in documentation is communicating our unique body of knowledge while demonstrating to the lay world that we are capable of providing effective and efficient patient care. This world includes not only purchasers but also other health care providers and individuals who read our reports. Through documentation we must demonstrate that we are competent to treat a patient with a specific diagnosis and are effective and cost efficient in doing so. We need to remember that in today's managed health care system the focus is on cost containment, and also on using the available resources to the best advantage to assure the best health outcome for society. This era demands results within given constraints.[6] It is apparent that now and in the future there will be need to make choices about the use of available resources. These choices will be based on the demonstrated effectiveness of different courses of treatment and increased competition among all providers for the limited resources. Dr. William Mohlenbrock[7] reinforced this view when he stated, "Quality providers [in his article he equated this to *effective* providers] deserve to receive the more profitable business; payers deserve to receive the value that results from the practice of high quality cost-efficient medicine, and the patient deserves nothing less!" If your documentation clearly demonstrates the direct line relationship between treatment intervention and functional limitation and also demonstrates that your treatment or intervention has changed the outcome for your patient, the effectiveness of your clinical decisions will be clearly demonstrated.

Let us examine one therapist's poor attempt to communicate his knowledge and effectiveness to both his referral sources and the payment source. To do that, consider a simple scenario: Dr. Hammer, a busy orthopedic surgeon, believes that *good*, aggressive rehabilitation is important to maintaining his reputation for getting patients well, but does not believe in owning his own rehabilitation practice. So Dr. Hammer sends the first patient referred from his new industrial client, Fabulous Furniture, to the new local physical therapy office. The referral reads, "evaluate and treat." This physician takes time to call the clinic and explain that the claimant began experiencing acute low back pain without referral below the knee after he lifted a single box weighing 100 lb from the floor to shoulder height at work. Six full weeks later Dr. Hammer's office received a note from the therapy clinic (Fig 2–5). Dr. Hammer read the notes and immediately uttered, "Oh my gosh! What is this therapist doing?" By reviewing the note he believes that this client was never evaluated and was immediately given a total regimen of *passive* modalities, something he definitely did not want to happen.

Now, let's shift our view to the office of Fabulous Furniture. The owner, Fanny Fab, decided last year to become self-insured for work-related injuries. She has been actively choosing providers for her injured workers based on their understanding of her needs and the needs of her injured employees. Just last month she finally selected an orthopedist, Dr. Hammer, after extensive review and discussion with him. She chose Dr. Hammer because

---

CLINICAL SUMMARY REPORT

Dear Dr. Hammer: Date: The present

Sam Stockboy is being seen in physical therapy for treatment of low back pain and myofascial dysfunction syndrome of the lumbar spine.

Treatment in the last 50 days: Hot packs and electrical stimulation to lumbar spine, paraspinal muscles, and gluteal musculature. Ultrasound to the bilateral lumbo-sacral thoracic areas, and both buttocks. Massage and myofascial release techniques to lower extremities with pelvic floor releases, manual therapy to lumbar spine, both SI joints. He also participates in biofeedback to decrease overuse of lumbar extensors while walking. We have recently switched from hot packs to cold packs to decrease inflammation. He was also issued a new TENS unit during this treatment series, which has four electrodes so patient can adequately cover the painful areas of thoraco-lumbo-sacral region extending into the bilateral buttocks and upper thighs. The one he recently purchased and has at home provides relief to a much smaller area.

Frequency of visits in last 50 days: Five times per week. Patient has missed some treatments during this series.

Assessment: Patient has progressed slowly during the first treatment series. He has increased muscle guarding and is not currently ambulating wel. He continues to present with extreme tenderness and muscle irritability.

Plan: Patient will continue to come to therapy for treatment as discussed above. Discussed with patient the importance of routine therapy. He stated that it is difficult for him.

Respectfully yours,

Master N. Motion, PT

cc: Fanny Fab
Fabulous Furniture
#2 U.R. Home Lane
W. Anytown,

FIG 2–5.
Note to a physician and the patient's employer imply a malingering patient and use of passive therapies.

she believed he would work with Fabulous Furniture *and* the injured employee to return the latter to maximum level of function as quickly as possible. This is important to Fanny because it is only in that way that the employee and Fabulous Furniture are in a win-win arrangement. Ms. Fab felt comfortable with Dr. Hammer and his referral to a physical therapist because she believed after reading his report that her injured employee was going to be shown techniques for independent pain control and then progress as rapidly as possible to a return-to-work program. Today, however, she saw the note in Figure 2–5. She can tell that her valued employee has been encouraged to receive physical therapy every day and has been doing so since the initial visit 6 weeks ago. She can also tell that her injured employee has *not* learned independent pain control, nor has his therapy progressed toward an early return to work. The information in the report contains no explanation she can understand about why the therapist believes it is necessary to schedule appointments so frequently or to continue to see the employee for so long, or why her key employee is spending *more than 2½ hours each day* receiving only passive treatments.

This leads to several questions. Does this note let the physician, Dr. Hammer in this case, or the self-insured employer, Fabulous Furniture and its owner Fanny Fab, see what a unique ability the treating physical therapist has to treat the patient effectively? *No!* Can either party make any sense of why the patient is being seen so often, what is being done, what kind of progress is being made, or when it will all end? *No!* What might the doctor and the employer think of this therapist, or indeed of all of physical therapy itself? The impression is that it is of no value and perhaps has even slowed the patient's recovery. This does not have to be the result of reporting or documenting.

Let us look at a different note on the same patient (Fig 2–6) and see if a different message is being conveyed.

As you can see, these notes do tell two different stories. They demonstrate clearly the unique perspective, ability, and effectiveness of physical therapy, and indeed of this physical therapist. It is important to emphasize that your documentation, or report writing, is the only way that any payer can make a determination of whether you receive any remuneration for the services you have provided. The way the care is documented should clearly demonstrate the clinical decision-making process as well as the effectiveness and efficiency of your clinical decisions in improving the outcome for your patient. If you have done this well, then the payer can easily make a positive determination.

Recognizing That Medical Records Are Widely Used as Business Records

In the business world, medical records are used by utilization review and management firms to make reimbursement decisions. Outpatient and inpatient rehabilitation reviews are conducted primarily as a means to reduce the total cost of health care. Until recently, reviews were most often conducted retrospectively by registered nurses or by technicians within the payers' own claims administration units.

CLINICAL SUMMARY REPORT

Dear Dr. Hammer: Date: The present

Sam Stockboy has been and is being seen in physical therapy at your request. He is being seen for the treatment of low back pain and myofascial dysfunction syndrome. Treatment began 50 days ago after his initial work-related injury. Onset of that injury followed a single lift of 100 lb from floor to shoulder height with a 45-degree twist to the left when weight was nearing maximum height. This is the first episode of low back pain for this man. It is important to note his complicating conditions of chronic obstructive pulmonary disease and morbid obesity. This patient's initial and current condition are detailed below:

	Initial	*Current*
Range of motion	Bilateral LE WNL	Bilateral LE WNL
	Thomas test showed marked iliopsoas shortening bilaterally	Thomas test negative
	Lumbar extension 10% range	Lumbar full extension/flexion
	Lumbar spine unable to forward flex beyond 30 degrees	Sidebend R full, L 7/8
	Side bend R full; L 1/4 range with spasm	Rotation R 7/8, L full
	Rotation R 1/4 range; L 3/4 range	
SLR	Negative bilaterally	Negative bilaterally
Manual Ms test:	Both LE's WNL	Both LE's WNL
	Rectus Abd 3+/5	Rectus Abd 4+/5
	Lower Abd 2/5	Lower Abd 4+/5
Walking tolerance:	15 ft followed by spasm of lumbar extensors	Min. 2,000 yd without spasm
	3 minutes on treadmill at 0 incline	35 minutes on treadmill at 6 mph at 0 incline
		25 minutes at 4.5 mph at 30 incline
Squatting ability:	Unable to squat from stand without pain	Squat from stand to floor maintaining normal posture and lifting 30 lb
	Unable to maintain normal curve	
Posture:	Markedly increased lumbar curve, with lateral shift to R; uneven weight bearing pattern R > L	Normal lumbar curve, slight lateral shift R; can self-correct in weight bearing

FIG 2–6.
Clinical summary report written to provide the physician and patient's employer with exact data on the initial assessment, current therapy, and patient prognosis.

Palpation:	Trigger point iliopsoas bilaterally	Normal
	Marked spasm L1–S3 paravertebrals	
Job duties:	Patient's job requires frequent squatting from stand and return to stand lifting weight up to 25 lb, two to five lifts from floor to shoulder with weight of 100 lb/day, and 7 to 8 hours of walking per day	

Treatment in the last 50 days:

Treatment began 50 days ago, with hot packs and electrical stimulation to lumbar paraspinals and gluteals to decrease spasm and increase circulation prior to treadmill and exercise for the first 14 days of treatment. Target for treadmill endurance based on minimum requirements of job. Patient also received ultrasound at 1.5 W/cm^2 to bilateral thoraco-lumbo-sacral region and both gluteals to promote tissue healing and decrease the inflammatory response. This was followed by manual therapy, active assistive correction of the right lateral shift, myofascial release technique of pelvic floor release, and deep iliopsoas work to decrease lumbar curve, improve normal LS posture, and decrease lateral shift. At day 10 and forward to present, this was complemented with extensive home stretching of iliopsoas and progressive abdominal and lower extremity exercises, detailed in the attached home exercise log sheet. Abdominal strength increased more than 20%, and a normal lumbar curve is now present in all positions required in job duties and activities of daily living. On treatment day 11 we switched to self-applied ice packs after the treadmill. At this time the patient was also instructed in, and is complying with, an aggressive home ambulation program (see attached log sheet to see progress from ambulation of one city block initially to current ambulation of up to 5 miles at an easy pace in the afternoon after therapy). Initial difficulty with ambulation was increased spasm of the paravertebrals, which did not respond to self-applied cold. A TENS unit with four electrodes was then initiated for home pain control with lengthy ambulation. Clinical approach for 2 weeks utilized a portable EMG biofeedback while the patient was ambulating on a treadmill until he could maintain musculature activity within acceptable limits.

Frequency of visits in the last 50 days: Five times per week. We have been seeing Mr. Stockboy to combine acute injury treatment with supervised work conditioning. The patient has missed three treatment sessions because of car trouble.

Assessment: Patient has progressed markedly, as seen by objective measures. He is, in my opinion, now able to meet requirements of Fabulous Fab's modified duty program, which he could begin on your release.

Plan: Patient to continue therapy before or after his modified work hours for work conditioning and supervision of his now independent pain control. Discussed with patient the importance of routine conditioning and correct posture.

Respectfully,

Master N. Motion, PT

FIG 2–6 (cont.).

Use of the registered nurse as a medical reviewer is a standard in the group insurance industry and in managed care. Nurse reviewers no doubt review the majority of claims. Unfortunately, there is no standard knowledge or experience level among this group. Many nurse reviewers are just out of school; others may have had extensive training in all aspects of medical care. In addition, some nurses may have years of experience and training in utilization review; others may have none. The nurse may also review in tandem with a board-certified utilization review physician. The experienced nurse reviewer expects to see physical therapy documentation that reflects the therapist's efforts to resolve any of the patient's problems in a timely manner and demonstrates concern for effective and efficient health care.

The technician is frequently used by Workers' Compensation companies to review claims as a part of claims administration. Training for the technician may be informal on-the-job training that covers interpretation of medical reports and claims determination, or it may include formal classroom instruction. Review of this course work reveals that there is no information on physical therapy services. The technician, even one with experience, will expect physical therapy documentation to present clearly what is wrong, how the therapist proposes to cure it, and how long it will take.

Regardless of the type of reviewer utilized, each payer creates a system to "flag" charts for evaluation of medical necessity or review. Common "flags" include the following:

- Excess treatment
- Excess duration
- Treatment inconsistency
- Chronicity
- A nonprofessional providing care
- No improvement
- Appropriateness of provider service
- No evidence of a "fading" schedule of treatment
- Continuous unmodified palliative modalities
- Lack of physical therapy documentation
- Lack of short term/long term goals
- Tests performed without report included
- Daily use of greater than three modalities
- Course of treatment not projected

Once a claim is flagged, what happens? Despite popular belief, usually no checklist is used to determine whether the services were appropriate and the bill should be paid. Overall, each reviewer first gets a general impression of services provided by reviewing the organization, legibility, and meaningfulness of the documentation that accompanies the bill. Because the medical reviewer cannot *see* the patient, conclusions about reimbursement must be based on clinical documentation and other available records. If the reviewer does not get your clinical documentation, he or she must base judgment only on your billing statements. And, as we know, no billing statement paints a complete picture of the patient's condition. When documentation or reports are available, medical reviewers make more favorable benefit and reimbursement determinations if the following information is included:

1. *Clearly identified problems:* The more functionally these problems are stated the more understandable they are to the medical reviewer.
2. *Reasonable treatment plan:* Based on your clearly identified patient problems the treatment plan makes sense. Don't expect the medical reviewers, even your peers to try to understand what you are doing. State it.
3. *Reasonable changes:* Patients do have complications that arise during treatment. Tell the medical reviewer.
4. *Reasonable results:* Physical therapists and all health care providers need to avoid the "till death do us part" treatment plan. The more professional the medical reviewer, the greater degree to which they will use professional and community standards of care to determine appropriateness.

The utilization review–claims review process is gradually changing. More and more medical and Workers' Compensation payers are contracting with outside companies to provide specialized review services, including peer reviews, for physical therapy claims. These services can include the traditional **retrospective review,** but often also include **prospective review** and **concurrent review.** The retrospective review process used by specialized reviewers is similar to the process previously mentioned. This review by peers would again develop recommendations for payments or denial on billings and the documentation that they have. The first area of focus for these reviewers is the relationship between noted dates of treatment and billing dates. Therefore it is important that bills and documentation correspond. Further recommendations of the reviewer are based on the correlation of your documentation with the *Standards of Practice* as set forth by the APTA (Appendix I–A) and the Practice Act of your state law. The degree to which you clearly identify the patient's problems, establish a reasonable, effective treatment plan, and carry it out is also of critical importance. Other areas of consideration include the appropriateness of your clinical decisions judged by research on efficiency of treatment, established physiologic response to treatment, and current standards of practice.

One of the recent moves within utilization review is the comparison of your documented clinical decision-making process with that of a set clinical algorithm (Fig 2–7). This comparison would again determine a reimbursement recommendation. In this case, the documentation of the process and results of your clinical decisions become critical and must reflect consideration of the important elements of care. Again, the fact that we must be writers, not just treaters, or not just thinkers, is evident.

We have been talking of utilization review and utilization management. However, as time passes, many purchasers are moving beyond these approaches to concepts of provider profiles. Evidence of this is revealed in the following quotes from *Business & Health* magazine by John Hanson, Direc-

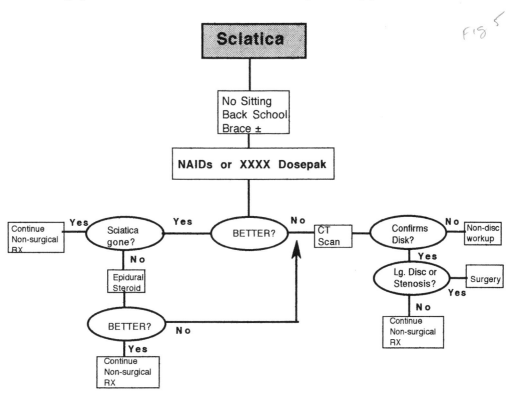

FIG 2–7.
Clinical algorithm in the form of a decision tree.

tor of Insurance for the Orange County, Florida, Public School System. Hanson suggests that when there is agreement on community standards (accepted standards of care for each diagnosis) and a method of accountability, the practitioners who meet those standards (i.e., who can demonstrate good effective outcomes and compliance with research-based community standards) will not have to submit to the typical utilization review (UR) practices prevalent today: "For those we trust, we can say 'You just practice medicine, send us the bill and we'll pay for it,' . . . but those who cannot perform up to those standards would still have to jump through UR Hoops!"

What are practice profiles, and how would you, as a practitioner, prove yourself enough that you can "just practice physical therapy"? Practice profiles are quite literally demonstrations and quantifications of the way you as a clinic or a practitioner practice that have been put in a database format. Most often the profiles are developed by reviewing your care and outcome by way of your bills and reports for a specific diagnosis or **ICD-9** code. The better profiles also have incorporated a factor into the calculations that indicates the severity of the patient's condition or co-morbidity or complicating factors. This profile is then compared with those of other providers within the same class for the same diagnosis and within the same geographic area. Examples of practice profiles for physicians are illustrated in Tables 2–2 through 2–4.

Table 2–2 shows a relatively simple comparison developed by an Independent Physicians Association to help educate physicians and to assist in contracting efforts. What you see in this profiling is a group of family practice physicians treating the same diagnosis who have all had the same result of their care: total relief of symptoms. Note the revisit rate and the average charge per patient. It should be obvious that given the same diagnosis and result, Dr. 4 has "proven" himself, and probably Mr. Hanson would tell him to "go practice medicine, send us the bill, and we'll pay for it."

Table 2–3 is information taken from a hospital, which is attempting to educate its medical staff and to determine which orthopedists were most effectively treating patients admitted with medical low back pain so that individual could head their new Industrial Medicine program. In this case the diagnosis was the same, DRG 243, and the result to be compared was "discharge from the hospital." Their standard for comparison was length of stay vs. the standard length of stay for that diagnosis established by Medicare. The information provided in the table was abstracted from billing information and patient records. To ease understanding, this data table was later translated into a graphic format. In this case, Dr. 33820 proved to be the most effective provider.

TABLE 2–2.

SUMMARY OF PHYSICIAN VISITS AND CHARGING PATTERNS*

Physician	Total Patients Seen	Patients Requiring Multiple Visits		No. of Multiple Visits	Average No. of Charges per Visit	Average No. of Visits per Patient	Total Charges (US Dollars)			Average Charge per Patient
		n	%				Primary Care Physician	Outside Lab, X-ray	All Charges	
M.D. 1	52	28	53.8	63	3.9	3.63	14,859.84	3,009.70	28,842.04	439.27
D.O. 2	26	17	65.4	31	2.1	3.15	5,687.00	154.00	5,991.00	230.42
M.D. 3	78	45	57.7	94	3.2	3.47	28,833.00	—		369.65
M.D. 4	122	25	20.5	42	1.4	2.15	11,088.00	599.20	12,084.25	98.54

*These data on sample practice patterns were developed by an Independent Physicians Association. They are summarized from charges submitted from January 1989 to the present.

TABLE 2–3.

INDEPENDENT PHYSICIAN PRACTICE PATTERN COMPARISON BY LENGTH OF STAY AND CHARGES FOR **DRG 243 (1989)**

Physician	DRG	Patient	Length of Stay (days)	Total Charges	Room Charges	Medicare Length of Stay (days)
32017	243	9280	9	$7,619.00	$2,205.00	5.3
	243	4998	12	$8,508.00	$2,920.00	5.3
	243	8369	6	$3,503.00	$1,500.00	5.3
	243	4747	11	$6,169.00	$3,025.00	5.3
Mean			9.5	$6,449.75	$2,412.50	5.3
33820	243	7925	1	$1,769.00	$ 275.00	5.3
	243	5297	6	$3,307.00	$1,500.00	5.3
Mean			3.5	$2,538.00	$ 887.50	5.3
33961	243	5180	6	$4,234.00	$1,350.00	5.3
	243	15	4	$2,631.00	$ 900.00	5.3
	243	95	6	$3,535.00	$1,470.00	5.3
	243	1341	2	$1,967.00	$ 450.00	5.3
	243	938	3	$2,344.00	$ 675.00	5.3
	243	1035	3	$2,319.00	$ 735.00	5.3
	243	1785	5	$4,050.00	$1,350.00	5.3
	243	2197	4	$3,337.00	$1,100.00	5.3
Mean			4.1	$3,052.13	$1,002.75	5.3

The final example is taken from the Workers' Compensation arena, and in this case the data profiles were used by the employer and insurer to determine which physicians would be designated to treat all of the company's work-related injuries. The information for these profiles was taken from billing information and a review of the Workers' Compensation medical file. This profiling not only looks at medical costs for DRG 215 (Fig 2–8) but also the larger associated cost of the injured employee's lost time (Fig 2–9).

Another interpretation of the provider profile is offered by a recent article in *Business Insurance*, which stated that "Employers need to realize you may have to pay more for the *right* providers instead of less. . . . Sometimes early expensive treatment can save money later on." Hanson expresses these views because he and many others active in the fight to contain costs believe that "discounts, utilization management, and other controls" have "maxed out" on effectiveness. He believes the biggest return on investment is in "state of the art computer systems, which could be used to gather and analyze medical data." This gathering and analysis of medical data, or use of outcome management techniques, is the next generation of utilization review. For the next 5 to 10 years we as providers will have to deal with both systems, so we must make documentation and reporting our best defense and offense in the upcoming struggles on the battlefield of managed care.

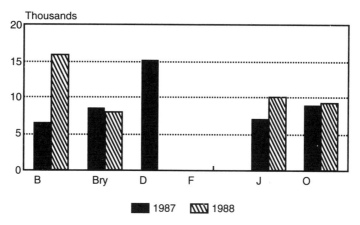

DRG 215   Total Charges

FIG 2-8.
Practice patterns in one orthopedic group.

LEGAL CONSIDERATIONS

Thus far in this chapter we have reexamined our practices and discussed at length the reimbursement considerations for our reporting. In addition, some of the basic tenets for reporting in today's health care environment have been addressed. Note, however, that documentation can also be reviewed for a legal claim. Although the idea is not attractive, avoiding legal issues would probably be disastrous. Therefore we must understand that documentation also *must be a legal document that displays a standard of care.*

Whether we like it or not, the practice of medicine, and as a result the practice of physical therapy, has become more litigious in the last decade. The fact that there has been an increase in frequency of **professional liability** claims as well as the increase in the size of awards and settlements for such claims (according to one physical therapy malpractice insurance company, the total cost for one case recently settled totaled over $780,000) is important for you to remember in all aspects of your practice, but is critical in your documentation habits. Your documentation and reports are legal records, and these legal records may be evidence for or against you in a professional liability case. Before further comment is made on documentation as a legal record, you as a therapist should understand the legal concept of

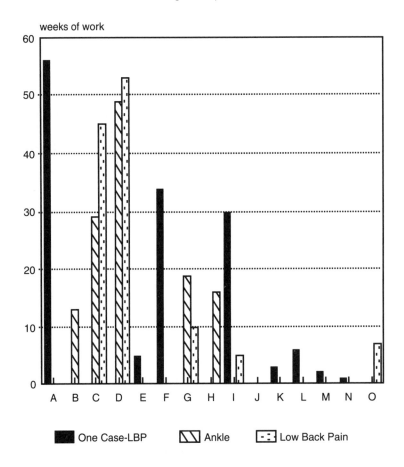

FIG 2–9.
Average lost time given by physician (diagnostic specific).

malpractice, the elements of malpractice, and what constitutes professional liability exposures.

Malpractice traditionally has been defined exclusively as **negligence** or *legally actionable careless treatment* resulting in injury to a patient.[8] However, for a suit by an injured patient to succeed, the patient must demonstrate that four major elements exist. The degree to which all four elements can be proved will determine the extent of malpractice when you are called to court or sued. One authority[9] states the major elements of malpractice as:

1. The physical therapist owed the patient a duty of care.
2. The physical therapist breached that duty of care.
3. The patient was injured.
4. This injury came about as a result of the physical therapist's breach of duty of care.

The first element is rarely important in any professional liability claim. The therapist, as a health care provider, is always considered to have a legal duty of care to the patient.

The second element is often viewed as the crux of a malpractice action. Violation of the required standard of care most closely compares to the general public's perception of "negligence." The question becomes, Did the therapist "breach" or deviate from the duty or **standard of care** that he or she owed the patient? Translated this means, Did the therapist evaluate and treat the patient according to an accepted "standard of care"? The critical factor here is, What is the expected standard of care? Authorities explain that the standards of care can be interpreted in two ways: by locality rule or by majority rule.

1. *Locality rule:* These standards are interpreted to mean that care given or in treatment of a particular type of ailment or injury should demonstrate the same standard of care given under like circumstances by therapy services in the *same* or *similar* localities.[9]

2. Majority rule: In this case, the treatment given must meet the standards of care *ordinarily* employed by members of the same profession.[9]

Locality rule has been largely abandoned, and replaced by majority rule.

What are the standards of care ordinarily employed by the physical therapy profession? Attorneys involved in medical malpractice cases frequently use appropriate state statutes, state and national legal decisions, and the standard of care developed and promulgated by the professional organization. In addition they use the testimony of known experts in that specific area of care to demonstrate the standard. Experts *do not* testify about what they *themselves* would have done under the circumstances. Experts testify as to whether the action of the therapist named in the suit passes as minimally acceptable clinical practice or meets the standard *ordinarily employed*. In each situation the standards that have been developed and promulgated by the professional organization are important. For physical therapy these are the *Standards of Care* developed by the House of Delegates of the APTA. A relevant excerpt from APTA Standards of Care is given in Table 2−4. The entire APTA Standards of Practice for Physical Therapy, as

TABLE 2–4.

STANDARDS OF CARE*

   X. *Informed Consent:*
      Physical therapist obtains the patient's informed
      consent in accordance with jurisdictional law
      before initiating physical therapy.
  XI. *Initial Evaluation:*
      Physical therapist performs and records an
      initial evaluation and interprets results to
      determine appropriate care for the individual.
  XII. *Plan of Care*
     1. Physical therapist establishes and records a
       plan of care for the individual, based on the
       results of the evaluation.
     2. Physical therapist involves the
       individual/significant other in the plan,
       implementation, and revision of the treatment
       program.
     3. Physical therapist plans for discharge of the
       individual, taking into consideration goal
       achievement, and provides for appropriate
       follow-up or referral.
 XIII. *Treatment*
     1. Physical therapist provides or delegates and
       supervises the physical therapy treatment
       consistent with the results of the evaluation
       and plan of care.
     2. Physical therapist records, on an ongoing
       basis, treatment rendered, progress, and
       change in status relative to the plan of care.
 XIV. *Reevaluation*
      Physical therapist reevaluates the individual
      and modifies the plan of care as indicated.

*From American Physical Therapy Association: *Standards of
Care.* Alexandria, Va, APTA, 1990. Used by permission.

well as the Guide for Professional Conduct and Code of Ethics and the APTA Policy Statement on Quality Assurance are given in Appendixes I–A to I–C.

Reviewing the Standards of Care, note that both the practice of physical therapy and the documentation of that practice are addressed. Because of this and the fact that report writing provides communication about the patient that can be critical, *failure to document accurately, clearly, and in a timely manner also constitutes negligence.* This failure may be the cause for a legal suit, dependent on the consequences of the omission. Suit for failure to communicate exists separate from any action based on quality of care rendered.[10]

What must you remember legally when you report? First, it is critical to remember that a medical record is admissible in court in malpractice and other legal proceedings. As part of your legal duty to any patient, you must provide accurate, complete, objective documentation of the patient's complaint(s), relevant history, evaluative findings, informed consent, and treatment. This documentation should clearly demonstrate that you, as the treating therapist, did not deviate from the standard of care ordinarily adhered to by the physical therapy profession, either in practice or in documentation of that practice. Therefore any patient record from your practice should include not only documentation of your daily treatment of that patient and his or her progress, but also an initial evaluation, with results interpreted so that an appropriate course of care is developed in conjunction with the individual (and/or significant other) and routine reevaluation and discharge planning are evident for this patient.

A secondary premise to remember when dealing with legal readers is that a *clear, concise, direct style conveys professional judgment and therefore acts as a strong defense.* Lack of the same can make your life a bit difficult.

Imagine that a professional liability suit has been filed against you and your practice. Despite the best efforts of your insurance company, all attempts at early settlement outside of court have failed. Now you are sitting in the cold hard seat of the witness stand. You hear the plaintiff's attorney mention your name and notice she is holding up a copy of your patient file on Jane Complainer, the claimant whom you first saw more than 5 years ago. As this scene is sinking into your senses, you pause to remember the first day you saw and evaluated Jane. It was a crazy, busy day. You had a new practice secretary who had scheduled five new patient evaluations for you before lunch. Ms. Complainer was number 4. By the time you began her evaluation she had been in the waiting room more than 40 minutes. You evaluated her neck pain symptoms quickly, running through a cursory range of motion evaluation, provided a muscle test, and then moved on quickly to the palpation part of your standard evaluation. You quickly decided she had experienced a simple cervical muscle strain of the upper trapezius and subscapularis. Consistent with the prescription you received to "evaluate and treat," you decided to use hot packs with high-voltage galvanic stimulation and deep tissue massage, to be followed by instruction in appropriate exercises. You used an assistant to complete the treatment while you went on to your next evaluation. That busy day ended quickly, and you had to leave without completing your documentation. "I will do it in the morning," you recall thinking. When morning came, details of the evaluation were a bit blurry. Were there any abnormal muscle grades? What did the sensory testing reveal? Did you do one? You charted as best you could, minimally, documenting only vague findings, and forgot the rest until today. You are roused

from your musing when the prosecuting attorney thrusts your initial evaluation under your nose and loudly demands, "Are you telling me, Ms.
Goodhands, that from this very specific [she uses this word "very" sarcasti-
cally] evaluation you can *really* determine Ms. Complainer's specific problem. That you really know enough to authorize a specific treatment plan for
her, which *of course* failed to take into account Jane's diabetes and her peripheral neuropathy?" As she states this last point, she flips on an overhead
projector and displays a *huge* copy of your initial and subsequent notes for
all the jury and the courtroom to see. You are completely at a loss. The adren-
aline is racing through your veins, your heart rate has far exceeded the 80%
of maximum you achieve in aerobics class, and you feel nauseous and without hope. The documentation that is now 20 times normal size on the courtroom wall is so vague and filled with illegible abbreviations that even you
can't see what you thought was wrong with Ms. Complainer. Why didn't
you note her diabetes, her neuropathy, and why did you give her only shoulder rolls as exercises. As you stare at your own horrid writing on the wall
and hear the tittling of the jurors, you realize you have no defense: your documentation has damned you. *Now* you know you *must modify* your approach to documentation. It needs to be clear and concise and explain *why*
what you found on evaluation needs to be treated in the way that you propose, and *what* you hope to achieve. You have found that *sloppy writing*, to
the jury and to all in that courtroom, indeed means sloppy thinking. This
situation is unfortunate, but one that could easily happen to you at the time
you least expect it. So prepare for it now by documenting clearly and concisely your evaluation, diagnosis, and treatment. Demonstrate your clinical
decision making clearly. Leave any reader, including the jury, a clear path
from what you found to what you did, why you did what you did, and the
result of any treatment.

   In addition to these strategies, which have been discussed at length, here
are some additional tips to follow when documenting or reporting, to create
a strong defense. Begin using these immediately, before it's too late!

- Always write on every line in the chart.
- Write with one pen. In the unusual case where a pen runs out of ink
  in the middle of an entry, indicate in a parenthetical note that the first
  pen ran out of ink.
- Correct mistakes by drawing a single line through the error and initial-
  ing (and dating, where required by law) the correction. Some attorneys
  advise that you also write "incorrect entry" by the error.
- Except for correcting contemporaneous mistakes, do not edit prior en-
  tries.

- Do not backdate an omission in the treatment record. Document any omitted prior entry as a new entry.
- Write legibly. Print if necessary.
- Do not express personal feelings about a patient (e.g., "Patient is a malingerer.").
- Do not argue with or disparage other health care providers within the record.
- Avoid including in the record extraneous verbiage not related to treatment.
- Avoid using terms or abbreviations not universally understood by all providers treating the patient.[10]

The last point to consider in understanding and dealing with your documentation or reporting practices from a legal perspective is that your reports *can* and *should* identify and provide necessary information for effective incident and risk management.

Even if you are the most successful physical therapist on this planet, there will probably be, in the course of your career, moments when your "perfection" results in an adverse incident. Again, documentation or reporting offers you an opportunity to collect and record all of the necessary information on this incident to protect yourself and manage your risks as a practitioner. To manage your risks, traditional risk management insists you begin by identifying these risks. This identification process can be the use of regular chart notes to indicate the occurrence of an adverse patient or visitor incident or the use of a special incident report. If you are using an incident report, it is important to separate the report from the patient's record to prevent discovery of this document by the opposing attorney. It is possible to limit this discovery according to APTA's *Risk Management Resource Guide* by preparing the report for an attorney. This *may* allow the incident report to then be considered privileged communication. It is recommended, however, that you discuss this with your attorney; it may depend on state statutes. Incident reporting should be done as soon as possible after any incident or adverse event has occurred. All staff should understand that the completion of an incident is NOT negative; rather, it serves to protect them. A sample incident/accident report is found in Appendix I–D.

Each physical therapy setting requires slightly different rules regarding the use of incident reports and the documenting of adverse incidents. Despite these differences, certain universal rules apply:

1. In *all* cases, when a physical therapist is aware of a potential incident, he or she should fully document the incident. The report should include the following:

   a. Identity of the patient.
   b. Complete description of the incident in objective terms.
   c. Where the incident occurred.
   d. When the incident occurred.
   e. Circumstances surrounding the incident.
   f. All potential witnesses to the incident.
   g. Any equipment the patient may have been using or working with at the time of the incident. Name of the manufacturer of the equipment.
   h. Actions taken to mitigate the injuries sustained by the patient as a result of the incident.
   i. All comments the patient may have made regarding the incident.
   j. Whether the patient may have somehow contributed to the injury.
2. Always document adverse incidents concisely and objectively. Do not speculate or assign blame in the record. Document as fact *only* what you personally sense.
3. Document as fact only what you experience personally.
4. What any person (including the patient or visitor) tells you about the situation that you did not personally observe, is *hearsay*[10] and should only be documented as *hearsay* (consult a dictionary for the meaning of *hearsay*). Hearsay is most easily documented as "*patient states* that the bedrail was left down by the physical therapist and that he fell out of bed when he rolled over. When the therapist entered room, it was observed that both head and foot bedrail were in full up position and pieces of patient's gown were caught between them."

   When and if a claim against the clinic, department, or therapist is made, the information from the incident report should be forwarded to the physical therapist's insurer and/or claim professional. In many cases it is useful to send this information to the insurer prior to notice of a lawsuit, as these statements and the investigation that the claims professional will conduct are useful tools in determining the liability of the therapist and perhaps mitigating the claim as well as developing and formulating a defense to the claim.

SUMMARY

   There are people outside our profession who control our destiny. These people, usually agents of the system and third-party payers, control the dollars we pay our staff, purchase new equipment, lease our space, and make a living by practicing our profession. Our survival requires us to work effectively within their constraints and to "break their resistance without fighting."

Our documentation and reporting have greatly influenced others' views of our profession and the ways they have chosen and will choose to control our moves and therefore our practices. Others' opinions of us are not all favorable; some, in fact, are severely negative. Such strong negative reactions to our reports, as presented earlier in this chapter, provide a clear signal that *now is the time to change and/or modify our approach to documentation*. We can no longer afford to "just do it."

Understanding who reads our reports is the first step to take in improvement. Once we understand who these powerful people outside our profession are, we can begin to get a sense of their thoughts, wants, and needs. From there we can relook at our practices and broaden our view of what that practice stands for. After doing these things, the fact is evident that we need to improve our documentation and reporting to include the following:

1. At initial patient contact:
   a. Clear statement of the problem(s), in terms understood by all readers and discussing the problem's effect on function.
   b. Plan of action that directly addresses the problem(s).
   c. Expected results, in terms of functional outcome, including how long the plan is going to take.
2. At interim points:
   a. Restatement of the initial problem.
   b. What you have done.
   c. Why you have done it.
   d. How it has been effective in changing the initial problem and function.
   e. How much longer will you need to treat the patient.
3. At patient discharge
   a. Restatement of the initial problem.
   b. What you have done.
   c. Why you have done it.
   d. How it has been effective in changing the initial problem and function.

In addition, we must remember these other critical considerations:

- Translating complex professional concepts into a form and language that can be understood easily by others outside the profession
- Clearly stating the problem or diagnosis in readily understandable terms

- Basing the treatment on resolving the problem identified and moving the patient to a specific functional result
- Providing a timeline for achieving that functional outcome or result through the treatment plan. If the plan is not effective in moving the patient toward that goal, frequent reevaluation and modification of the initial plan are expected.
- Clearly demonstrating the therapist's unique capability when dealing with each specific problem or diagnosis and demonstrating the efficacy of our treatment approach.
- Recognizing that medical records are widely used as business records and sources of information by insurance companies as well as utilization review/management firms.

The people who control our destiny are not only in the purchaser arena; individuals in a variety of legal professions also exert powerful influences over our practice. Although our natural tendency is to avoid "legal eagles," avoiding them, like avoiding reimbursement issues, would probably be disastrous.

It is time to improve our standard practice, to move to clear concise documentation that takes us beyond reporting impairments in PT-ese. Improvement will take us to a new way to communicate, a new way to break free of our struggle. It takes us to a place where we have survived the battle, survived the war, and are flourishing in a new peace with the systems outside us. The way to move to this better plane is by reporting functional outcomes through a logical clinical decision-making model.

REFERENCES

1. Sun Tzu: *The art of war,* James Clavell, editor, New York, 1983, Dell, pp 14, 17, 18.
2. Taulbee P: Outcomes management: buying value and cutting costs, *Business & Health,* March 1991, p 28.
3. Hubbard, DD: Views, *Healthweek,* August 12, 1991, p 17
4. Lewis B, Pucelik F: *Magic demystified: a pragmatic guide to communication and change,* Portland, Ore, 1982, Metamorphous Press.
5. American Physical Therapy Association Board of Directors Policies, Model definition of physical therapy for state practice acts, 03-86-22-85. Alexandria, Va, 1985, APTA.
6. Mooney G: *Economics: the road to better physiotherapy,* London, 1991, World Confederation for Physical Therapy.
7. Mohlenbrock WC: *Front Health Services Management* 1989; 5:4.

8. Scott RW: The legal standard of care, *Clin Management*, March/April 1991.

9. Harker RC: Malpractice and Other Bases of Potential Liability for the Physical Therapist, 5.1—Risk Management, An APTA Malpractice Resource Guide, Alexandria, Va, APTA.

10. Scott RW: Legal aspects of documenting patient care, *Phys Ther Today*, Summer 1991, pp 18–23.

TEST YOUR KNOWLEDGE

1. "Quality" physical therapy has many meanings. List seven different perceptions of the meaning of quality, and highlight at least three that are payor based.

2. Explain what V = Q/C means in terms of an employer's approach to health care.

3. What you write and how you write influences others' opinions of your capability and that of the profession. Name at least five types of readers of our notes, and briefly compare and contrast their expectations of our reporting.

4. Summarize and in clear terms state the key elements of an initial report and any interim report from the payer's perspective.

5. Complex physical therapy concepts must be translated. Provide two examples of "translation" of findings into assessment and then onto treatment. These examples should not be those found in the book.

6. Why must the reporting we do base our treatment on resolving the identified problem and moving toward a functional result?

7. List five of the common "flags" for medical review of a physical therapist's bill, then describe the information needed on claims submission to improve chances for favorable benefit and reimbursement terminations.

8. Compare and contrast retrospective review, prospective review, concurrent review, and practice/provider profiles. Further describe the trend with review, if there is one, or "the trend you see."

9. Malpractice traditionally has been defined exclusively as _____ or _____. What four elements must be proved to determine if malpractice exists?

10. What is the current interpretation of "standard of care"? How is this determined?

11. List five general legal rules for documentation, and explain why they are important.

12. Incident reporting is a critical part of the risk management and documentation process. Detail at least five universal rules for incident reporting, and explain why they are important.

TEST YOUR KNOWLEDGE ANSWER SHEET

1. Any of the following is acceptable.
   a. Care provided by a clinician who has participated routinely in professional development experiences
   b. Care that generates therapist or staff satisfaction
   c. Care provided by the same therapist or practitioner
   d. Care that meets the standard of care in my community or region or nationally
   e. Care that adds to the general well-being of the patient
   f. Care that provides symptomatic relief to the patient
   g. Care that meets or exceeds patient expectations for the treatment
   h. Care that generates patient satisfaction
   i. Care that meets key customer satisfaction issues for the patient
   j. Care that effects complete resolution of the objective findings
   k. Care that leads to improved clinical outcome
   l. Care that leads to a quantifiable functional improvement
   m. Care that generally improves the health status of the patient
   n. Care that is appropriately and completely documented
   o. Care that leads to quantifiable functional improvement within the limits of reimbursement
   p. Care that lowers the total work days lost due to injury or illness
   q. Care that makes the maximum possible contribution to the reduction of lost productivity
   r. Care that is cost efficient

2. $V = Q/C$ (value = quality divided by cost) is the method many purchasers of health care have used within the past 15 years. During the 1980s these purchasers vigorously pursued decreasing the cost of health care with questionable value to increase the value of their dollars spent. This was done through many types of discounting arrangements. However, health care inflation continued. Late in 1988 the other part of the equation, that is, quality, began to become important. Quality did not mean care provided by the same therapist or in a clinic within a JCAHO-accredited facility; instead, quality was examined through outcome management care, which led to quantifiable functional improvement within the limits of reimbursement. Care was considered in terms of being effective and efficient. The early 1990s have seen an increasing number of employers move toward selection of providers by assessment of their outcomes.

3. Any of the following:

Primary and referring physicians

Physician's nursing staff

Other physical therapists

Occupational therapists

JCAHO representatives

CARF representatives

Utilization review nurses

Utilization review physicians

Technicians involved in claims review

Preferred Provider Organization staff

Physical therapy peer review companies

State examining committee staff

Fraud investigators

Social services staff

Discharge planners

Home health agencies

Workers' Compensation technicians

Workers' Compensation claims adjusters

Workers' Compensation supervisors

Workers' Compensation auditors

Group health claims representatives

Group health claims auditors

Medical bill review service staff

Auditing firms

Malpractice defense attorneys

Malpractice defense attorney's staff

Malpractice plaintiff attorneys

Malpractice plaintiff attorney's staff

Jury members

Judges

Expert witnesses for the defense

Expert witnesses for the plaintiff

Potential expert witnesses for either side

HMO staff

Medicare intermediary review nurses

Medicare intermediary review therapists

Preferred Provider Organization utilization review

Physical therapy preferred providers

Utilization review team members

4. a. Initially needed is:
    (1) A clear statement of the problem(s), in terms understood by all readers and discussing the problem's effect on function
    (2) A plan of action that directly addresses the problem(s)
    (3) The expected result, in terms of function, including how long the plan is going to take
    b. Interim reports needed
    (1) A restatement of the Initial Problem
    (2) A statement of what you have done
    (3) A statement of why you have done that
    (4) A statement of how your action has been effective in changing the initial problem and function

(5) A declaration of how much longer you will need to treat the patient

5. The two examples should be similar to the following:

Assessment of functional limitations	**Translate to** $\longrightarrow$	**Treatment**
Patient is unable to:	○ ○ ○ ○ ○ ○	Needs home exercise program that
Elevate right arm past		includes _____
shoulder		Needs shoulder mobilization, e.g., __
Therefore unable to perform		_____
work duties		Needs modified work, e.g., _____
		_____

6. The knowledge base of payers and their representatives regarding clinical decision making is minimal; therefore the process and the rationale that lead you as clinician through the process is critical to ensure payment.
7. Any of the following:
   a. Excess treatment
   b. Excess duration
   c. Treatment inconsistency
   d. Chronicity
   e. Non-professional signs
   f. No improvement
   g. Appropriateness of provider service
   h. No evidence of a "fading" schedule of treatment
   i. Continuous unmodified palliative modalities
   j. Lack of physical therapy documentation
   k. Lack of short term/long term goals
   l. Tests performed without report included
   m. Daily use of greater than three modalities
   n. Course of treatment not projected

As we know, no billing statement paints a complete picture of the patient's problem. If possible, documentation or reports should be made available to their viewer, and should include the following information:
   a. Clearly identified problems. The more functionally these problems are stated the more understandable they are to the medical reviewer.
   b. Reasonable treatment plan. Based on your clearly identified patient problems the treatment plan makes sense. Don't expect the medical reviewers, even your peers, to "try to understand" what you are doing. State it.
   c. Reasonable changes. Patients do have complications that arise during treatment. Tell the medical reviewer. Remember, their crystal ball is in the shop!

    d. Reasonable results. Physical therapists and all health care providers need to avoid the "til death do us part" treatment plan. The more professional the medical reviewer the more they will use professional and community standards of care to determine appropriateness.

8. a. *Retrospective review:* A review of medical care the patient received after the care has been provided to determine if the services provided were appropriate and medically necessary. This determination is often made by review of billing statements, charting, reports.

    b. *Prospective review:* A approval process used to determine if proposed medical care treatment to be provided is medically necessary and/or appropriate for that diagnosis or *prior to* the rendering of the care.

    c. *Concurrent review:* Traditionally used to define a review that occurs at the same time as the medical care is given. This type of review is frequently seen as a way to evaluate length of stay, appropriateness of services, and discharge planning for patients in acute care facilities, but may also be applied to review of care in other settings.

    d. *Practice/provider profiles:* The utilization review/claims review process is gradually changing from one that is retrospective based to more prospective-concurrent review. There have been recent moves toward comparison of documented clinical decision making against an algorithm. In recent years, the purchasers have gone beyond even these approaches to managing utilization through comparison of provider profiles. These profiles are data-based demonstrations of how you practice.

9. *Negligence, legally actionable careless treatment*

    a. The physical therapist owed the patient a duty of care.

    b. The physical therapist breached that duty of care.

    c. The patient was injured.

    d. Injury was due to the physical therapist's breach of duty of care.

10. *Majority rule.* In this case, the treatment given must meet the standards of care *ordinarily* adhered to by members of the same profession. Attorneys involved in medical malpractice cases frequently use the standard of care developed and promulgated by the professional organization, and in addition use the testimony of known experts in that specific area of care to demonstrate the standard. Experts do not testify about what they themselves would have done under the circumstances. Experts testify as to whether the action of the therapist indicated in the suit passes as minimally acceptable clinical practice or meets the standard ordinarily adhered to. In each situation the standards that have been developed

and promulgated by the professional organization are important. For physical therapy these are the *Standards of Care* developed by the House of Delegates of the APTA.

11. Any of the following:
    a. Always write on every line in the chart.
    b. Write with one pen. In the unusual case in which a pen runs out of ink in the middle of an entry, indicate parenthetically that the first pen ran out of ink.
    c. Correct mistakes by drawing a single line through the error and initialing (and dating, where required by law) the correction.
    d. Except for correcting contemporaneous mistakes, do not edit prior entries.
    e. Do not backdate an omission in the treatment record. Document any omitted prior entry as a new entry.
    f. Write legibly. Print if necessary.
    g. Do not express personal feelings about a patient (e.g., "Patient is a malingerer.").
    h. Do not argue with or disparage other health care providers in the record.
    i. Avoid including extraneous verbiage not related to treatment in the record.
    j. Avoid using terms or abbreviations not universally understood by all providers treating the patient.
12. Any of the following:
    a. In *all* cases, when a physical therapist is aware of a potential incident, he or she should fully document the incident. The report should include:
       (1) Identity of the patient.
       (2) Where the incident occurred.
       (3) When the incident occurred.
       (4) Circumstances surrounding the incident.
       (5) All potential witnesses to the incident.
       (6) Any equipment the patient may have been using or working with at the time of the incident
       (7) Name of the manufacturer of the equipment.
       (8) Actions taken to mitigate the injuries sustained by the patient as a result of the incident.
       (9) All comments the patient may have made regarding the incident.
       (10) Whether the patient may have somehow contributed to the injury.

  b. Remember, it is important to document any incident concisely and objectively.

      (1) Always document adverse incidents concisely and objectively. Do not speculate as to fault in the record. Document as fact *only* what you personally sense.

      (2) It is important not to speculate or to assign blame within the record.

      (3) Document as fact only what you experience personally.

      (4) What any person (including the patient or visitor) tells you about the situation that you did not personally observe is hearsay and should only be documented as hearsay.

  c. Hearsay is most easily documented as "*patient states* that the bedrail was left down by the PT and he fell out of bed when he rolled over. When therapist entered room, it was observed that both head and foot bedrail were in full up position and pieces of patient's gown were caught between them." Incident/occurrence reports offer you an opportunity to collect and record all necessary information on an incident to protect yourself and manage your practice.

Building Documentation Using a Clinical Decision-Making Model

Bette Ann Harris, M.S., P.T.

Key Concepts

- Rationale for the model
- Model of orthopedic dysfunction
- Applying the model
- Case study

RATIONALE FOR THE MODEL

Effective documentation must be based on organized information and should reflect sound, justified physical therapy care. It is recognized that organized systems of note writing systematically guide the therapist to record key information in a time efficient manner. However, to consistently produce effective documentation, clinicians must be able to explain why they chose a particular examination or treatment or interpreted signs and symptoms in a certain manner. Understanding the cause of dysfunction is essential to the clinical decision-making process that occurs prior to establishing and documenting the prognosis, duration, and frequency of treatment. Because of this necessity, there has recently been interest in developing clinical decision-making models that guide the clinician in developing specific, logical treatment programs based on analysis of the patient's problem, subjective and objective findings, and realistic treatment goals. Several models have been developed and are being incorporated into educational programs and clinics across the United States. One such model is the model of orthopedic dysfunction for clinical decision making in physical therapy practice.[1]

The model is offered as a guideline for therapists (1) to assist them as they formulate and compare a hypothesis of dysfunction and (2) to provide a foundation for the clinician in presenting an appropriate and acceptable rationale for treatment in their documentation. This model is helpful in organizing the data gathered into a cohesive, understandable note that can be read by other caregivers and third-party payers to evaluate the standard of care.

In this chapter, the model of orthopedic dysfunction is presented first, followed by a sample case study and sample documentation using this decision-making strategy. The emphasis of the case presentation is to illustrate the use of the model for documentation, not to discuss treatment strategies. For readers interested in alternative models of clinical decision analysis, we refer you to the July 1989 issue of the journal *Physical Therapy*.[1]

MODEL OF ORTHOPEDIC DYSFUNCTION

The model of orthopedic dysfunction was developed to present a unifying framework of pathophysiologic and pathokinesiologic processes to illustrate theoretically the development of orthopedic dysfunction and its effects. The model is based on the static and dynamic properties and function of the neuromusuloskeletal tissues and structures.[2-11] The altered properties of these tissues are related to the cause and development of pain, impairment, functional limitations, and disability. We believe that by linking all of these elements together the clinician will be able to generate treatment hypotheses, develop more precise treatment programs, and analyze their results based on the patient's dysfunction. We recognize that other contributing variables, such as the psychologic, social, and functional needs of patients, strongly influence treatment strategies and therapy outcome. These other variables (not addressed here) also need to be examined and evaluated when writing a physical therapy assessment.

The model expands on the classic concept of a stimulus causing a response. The major sequence of events leading to the development of functional limitations, disability, and handicap are listed as follows:

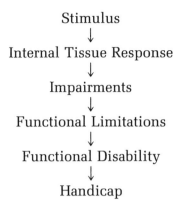

Although this particular chain of events will not apply in all patients, it is true in most clinical situations. Figure 3–1 details those stimuli and subsequent internal tissue responses that theoretically result in orthopedic dysfunction. Although all sections of the figure could be expanded, we have chosen to diagram the internal response section in the most detail to allow clinicians to analyze the patient's impairments and disabilities based on the pathophysiology of the dysfunction.

Terminology

Before we examine the model and its application, it is helpful to review its terminology. Impairments, functional disability, and handicap have been defined by the World Health Organization (WHO),[12] and *functional limitation* by Nagi.[13] **Impairments** refer to abnormalities of anatomic, physiologic, or psychologic origin within specific organs or systems of the body. Physical therapists tend to evaluate or measure impairments, for example, decreased range of motion, limited muscle performance, and altered sensation. Furthermore, many physical therapy interventions are targeted at alleviating or reducing the patients impairments and not the functional limitations. **Functional limitations** are restrictions or inability to perform activities of daily living (ADL) skills such as transfers, gait, and bed mobility. These limitations are the pieces that make up the functional disability that we as physical therapists can measure and also target part of our treatment interventions in lessening or alleviating these limitations. **Functional disability** refers to restriction of or inability to perform a normal range of ADL. WHO has classified functional disability into four categories: physical, mental, social, and emotional. Examples of physical disabilities we all deal with as physical therapists are limitations of ADL, such as inability to walk, and

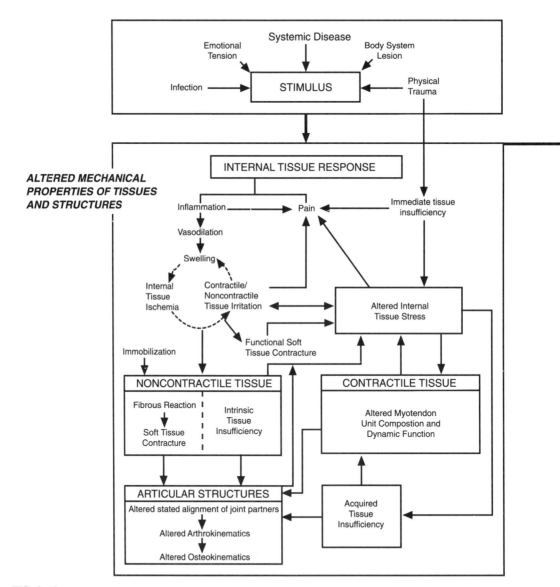

FIG 3–1.
Model of orthopedic dysfunction and its implications for examination and treatment. (Adapted from Harris BA, Dyrek DA: *Phys Ther* 69:548–553, 1989.)

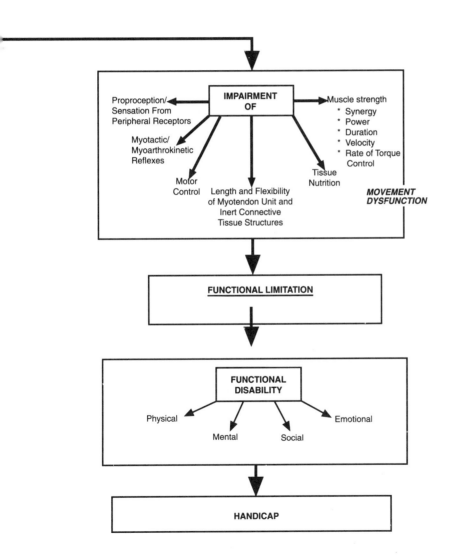

higher level activities, such as inability to participate in athletic games. **Handicap,** a much broader term, describes limitations in the fulfillment of a person's normal role, depending on age, sex, and social and cultural factors. An example of a handicap is inability to perform one's occupation. (A sample listing of WHO classifications of ambulation disabilities and skeletal impairments appears in Appendix II—A, and definitions in the Glossary.) The authors of this model have selected this terminology because it enables the clinician to differentiate between the impairment, the functional limitations, and subsequent disability.

APPLYING THE MODEL

Application of the Model of Orthopaedic Dysfunction requires linkage between the internal response of the tissue, the impairment, and the functional limitation. The important aspect of clinical decision making is selecting the correct therapeutic intervention. To make this selection the intervention must be related to the cause of the dysfunction; if not, the intervention is likely to address only the impairment side of the model.[1] These linkages must also be reflected in documentation, because they provide the rationale for treatment. By reviewing the events that occur in the internal tissue response section of the model the clinician can formulate a hypothesis of dysfunction by identifying the phases of reaction of the involved tissues. Once this hypothesis is formulated the clinician can propose more sensitive treatment techniques based on the altered tissue properties, then more appropriately demonstrate, through documentation, the clinical interventions.[1]

We have also developed generic treatment goals that parallel the sequence outlined in the internal tissue response section and in the impairments, functional limitations, and disability sections of the model:

1. Promote healing by improving the nutritional status of soft tissue
2. Prevent abnormal soft tissue flexibility and length for contractile and noncontractile tissues or restore normal flexibility and length
3. Prevent the loss of normal joint alignment or restore normal joint alignment
4. Prevent the loss of normal joint mobility or restore normal joint mobility
5. Promote normal myoarthrokinetic reflexes
6. Promote normal motor control
7. Promote normal cardiopulmonary and cardiovascular status
8. Decrease pain and associated symptoms

9. Prevent recurrence of lesion
10. Improve patient's functional status

These generic goals are based on the events outlined in the internal Tissue response section; appropriate interventions are determined by certain events that have taken place or should be prevented. The therapist needs to determine the appropriate goals based on information gathered during the interview process and subsequent examination of the patient. We have found these generic goals to be useful in guiding treatment choices based on the analysis of the dysfunction. Application of these generic goals to analyze specific orthopedic dysfunctions is outlined as follows:

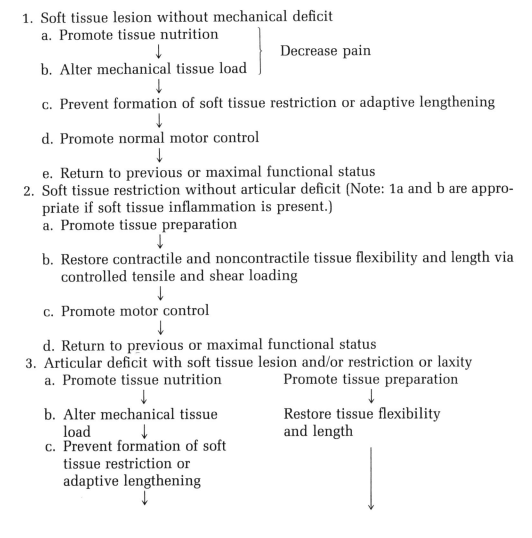

1. Soft tissue lesion without mechanical deficit
   a. Promote tissue nutrition
   b. Alter mechanical tissue load ⎫ Decrease pain
   c. Prevent formation of soft tissue restriction or adaptive lengthening
   d. Promote normal motor control
   e. Return to previous or maximal functional status
2. Soft tissue restriction without articular deficit (Note: 1a and b are appropriate if soft tissue inflammation is present.)
   a. Promote tissue preparation
   b. Restore contractile and noncontractile tissue flexibility and length via controlled tensile and shear loading
   c. Promote motor control
   d. Return to previous or maximal functional status
3. Articular deficit with soft tissue lesion and/or restriction or laxity
   a. Promote tissue nutrition   Promote tissue preparation
   b. Alter mechanical tissue   Restore tissue flexibility
      load   and length
   c. Prevent formation of soft
      tissue restriction or
      adaptive lengthening

(1) Restore proper static joint alignment
$\downarrow$ $\downarrow$
(2) Restore normal joint mobility
$\downarrow$ $\downarrow$
(3) Restore normal motor control
$\downarrow$

d. Return to previous or maximal functional status

CASE STUDY

In this section a case study is used to describe how to use the model for effective documentation.

History of Present Problem

Carol is a right-handed 34-year-old medical secretary who was referred to physical therapy for examination and treatment of her right knee. Carol sustained an injury to her right knee while skiing on February 10, 1990. She reported that while traversing to the left, her right knee hit hard in mid-flexion onto a mogul, and she felt her knee "jam together" as in a vise. Carol reports that she had immediate and severe pain, making it impossible for her to continue to ski down the mountain. She was brought to the base of the mountain on a toboggan and immediately examined by a physician. He immobilized her right knee in a long leg splint, and recommended the use of ice and of anti-inflammatory drugs. Carol was unsure of what the diagnosis was at that time, but she "knew it was serious and she probably would require surgery."

Carol was seen 3 days later by an orthopedic surgeon at the hospital where she is employed. The examination revealed that Carol was unable to weight bear on the right lower extremity and had effusion (3+) on the right knee. Passive range of motion was 10 to 50 degrees. Results of the Lachman's test were 2−3+ (anterior drawer in 20 degrees of flexion) with a soft end point, and there was tenderness along the lateral joint line and medial epicondyle of the right knee. There was also valgus laxity at 30 degrees, with a soft, painful end point. Radiographs were within normal limits. Magnetic resonance imaging revealed a right torn anterior cruciate ligament (ACL) and an avulsed medial collateral ligament from the tibia. The orthopedic surgeon recommended immediate surgical repair and reconstruction.

Carol's right knee was surgically repaired on February 23, 1990. The operative note read: "Right ACL replacement using doubled loop semitendinosus tendon transfer (arthroscopic assist); repair of tibial (medial) collateral ligament (open)." Carol's right lower extremity was placed in a Bledsoe brace in full extension for immobilization. She began ambulating with crutches and the brace

4 days postoperatively, with a touch-down gait. Knee range of motion exercises were initiated 3 weeks after surgery, and the brace was unlocked at that time to permit 0–90 degrees range of motion. Follow-up examination of the right knee by a physician on April 9, 1990, revealed 5 to 25 degrees of right knee flexion, moderate knee effusion, and pain. Referral for physical therapy was made at that time, and Carol was seen by a physical therapist the next day, April 10, 1990.

Carol's past medical history was noncontributory. She had no history of previous injuries, trauma, or serious illnesses. The only medications she used were anti-inflammatory drugs for pain and swelling of her right knee.

Social.—As previously stated, Carol works as a medical secretary. She is happily married and lives in a second floor (no elevator) condominium. Carol is normally very active: she skis, plays tennis, and attends aerobic classes three to five times per week. Carol was highly motivated to be able to return to her athletic activities.

Initial Physical Therapy Examination

Subjective: Carol complained that her knee felt very stiff and that she was unable to walk comfortably. She reported that she had difficulty putting weight on the right leg.

Inspection: The right knee was moderately swollen (2+ effusion), and there was extra-articular soft tissue swelling. The knee was reddish blue. There were also well-healed medial and lateral incisions and several arthroscopic incisions.

Palpation: There was moderate pain along the lateral incision and along the lower third of the patella tendon

Range of motion: There was 5–30 degrees of knee flexion (sitting), active assisted only. Patella mobility was restricted in all directions (grades 1 and 2).

Special tests: None were performed at the time.

Strength and motor control:
    All uninvolved extremities and trunk: 5/5
    (R) hip: grossly 3+/5
    (R) knee: quad set 2/5
    (R) knee flexion: 2+/5
    (R) ankle: grossly 3/5

Function: Patient presently walking with crutches, with weight bearing as tolerated on right lower extremity. Wearing Bledsoe brace unlocked (0–90 degree flexion). Not working or driving. No athletic activities.

Now that you have read the case, you are probably thinking that this patient presents the clinician with a fairly straightforward physical therapy plan and subsequent treatment program. However, unless care is appropriately justified through documentation of your clinical decision making, the prognosis, frequency, and duration of the treatment program may well be scrutinized by third-party payers. Analyzing this case study using the Model of Orthopaedic Dysfunction can serve to substantiate the need for physical therapy.

Tables 3–1 and 3–2 highlight the key information obtained from reading this case study. Carol's most important functional disability at this time is that she is unable to walk without crutches, which limits her activities enough that she cannot manage her daily routines. To put this in terms of functional limitations, she is unable to walk without pain and stiffness, and cannot fully bear weight on the right lower extremity.

Now you need to ask yourself, What impairments are contributing to her functional limitations? These include decreased range of motion in her right knee, pain, swelling, and decreased strength in her right lower extremity. The next step of the analysis is to review the internal tissue response section of the model and determine which of these impairments are amenable to physical therapy, and decide how long you expect it will take to resolve these problems. Figure 3–2 highlights the key information to be considered in making these decisions. We can hypothesize that the severely restricted patellofemoral mobility is a side effect of the healing process and the long period of immobilization. The limited osteokinematic motion of the tibiofemoral joint also results from these same causes, and is complicated by knee effusion. We also know that muscle weakness is caused by disuse and that the quadriceps muscle is further inhibited by swelling.[14, 15] The knee was surgically reconstructed approximately 6 weeks previously, so we also know

TABLE 3–1.

INITIAL EVALUATION: RIGHT KNEE

Impairment: Decreased range of motion, 5°–80°
Functional limitation: Inability to ambulate without pain and stiffness
Functional disability: Unable to carry out normal activities of daily living

Impairment	Method of Evaluation	Results
Increased temperature and effusion	Temperature testing by palpation Girth measurement	Warm joint Girth 2–3 inches larger than left knee
Limited patellofemoral and tibial glide	Accessory mobility testing	Decreased mediocaudal patellar glide Decreased mediotibial glide
Decreased soft tissue extensibility	Positional testing Palpation	Decreased range of motion
Altered firing pattern of right quadriceps; right lower extremity weakness	Quadriceps set at 10° (with towel roll)	Reflex inhibition of quadriceps muscle

TABLE 3–2.

TREATMENT PLAN: RIGHT KNEE

Initial Problem	Treatment Goals	Specific Techniques
Increased effusion	Decrease effusion so that knee temperature and girth are same as in left knee	Electromuscular stimulation (low pulse rate) Ice Compression
Decreased tibiopatellar glide	Increase patellar mobility	Mobilization of patella (grade 1–3 as tolerance improves)
Decreased soft tissue extensibility	Increase extensibility of quadriceps, hamstring, and gastrocnemius muscles	Massage Stretching exercises
Decreased range of motion, 5°–80°	Achieve 5°–120° range of motion with normal arthrokinematics and osteokinematics	Joint mobilization Proprioceptive neuromuscular facilitation Therapeutic exercises

that this knee is undergoing the healing process and that tissue at this time is fairly weak. Therefore any techniques chosen to increase range of motion must not be so vigorous as to disrupt the healing repair. Strengthening at this time will be nonproductive because of the knee effusion, and could be potentially negative given the newness of the surgical repair.

Therefore the treatment goals, in order of priority; should be

1. To decrease the knee effusion, which should decrease the pain
2. To increase patellofemoral mobility, which will contribute to increased tibiofemoral motion
3. To increase strength of the right lower extremity, which should be achieved as the other problems resolve

The long-term goal is to increase weight-bearing ability and improve gait so that functional limitations can be resolved.

The time-line for treatment will be dependent on the response to therapy, the environment, and the patient's previous functional level. The patient who has undergone an uncomplicated surgical knee reconstruction should regain full function at approximately 1 year postoperatively. However, ongoing frequent physical therapy would not be needed. Once Carol has regained normal knee range of motion and has a normal gait pattern at full weight bearing, most of the exercises can be continued as a home program with supervision. If, however, she were a high-level athlete and her functional goal was to return to competition, the knee would need to be rehabilitated to a higher level of fitness. By continually relating the impairments, functional limitations, and disability to each other and to the pa-

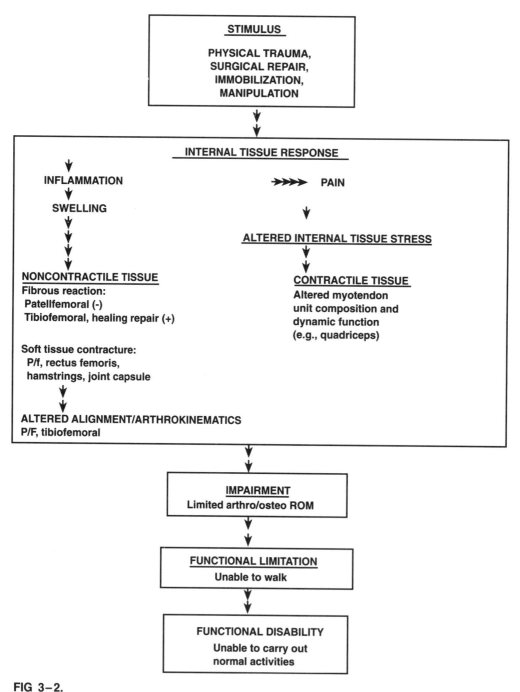

FIG 3–2.
Factors limiting range of motion. These factors can be viewed in terms of the model presented in Figure 3–1.

tient's environment and/or previous level of functioning, the need for physical therapy can be substantiated through documentation.

Now suppose that after the initial evaluation was done and the treatment goals outlined, the treatment to decrease the effusion and increase range of motion yielded no change. In fact, any attempt to increase range of motion resulted in increased pain, swelling, and no change in motion. This should lead you to ask yourself why? There could be two potential reasons: (1) The physical therapy is inappropriate (e.g., wrong choice of techniques, too vigorous) or, assuming that the patient is compliant and cooperative. (2) Something else is going on physiologically. Careful review of the physical therapy treatment plan and review of the internal response section of the model should lead you to the correct analysis. Perhaps the patient should be referred back to the surgeon for further testing (e.g., to rule out low-grade infection or excessive adhesion formation).

This case is a good illustration of how the same "diagnosis" and problems can lead to different courses of physical therapy, each with markedly different durations of treatment. The therapist can use the model to help identify the various courses of treatment results in a particular patient during physical therapy. Because third-party payers are more vigorously reviewing and monitoring physical therapy, it is of utmost importance that physical therapists be able to clearly justify both the type and the duration of care patients receive. This course of preparation is necessary to provide the best care possible for each patient.

Now that you have reviewed this model of critical decision making,* we need to turn our attention to the next extension of functional outcome assessment, that is, documentation of functional outcome. As you read Chapter 4, which outlines a particular note-writing strategy, we suggest you apply this decision-analysis process when determining the critical pieces of information to include in your documentation.

REFERENCES

1. Harris BA, Dyrek DA: A model of orthopaedic dysfunction for clinical decision making in physical therapy practice, *Phys Ther* 69:548–553, 1989.
2. Akeson WH, Dip DA: Effects of immobilization on joints, *Clin Orthop* 219:28–36, 1986.
3. Brooks VB: Motor control: how posture and movements are governed, *Phys Ther* 63:664–673, 1983.
4. Cailliet R: *Soft tissue pain and disability*, Philadelphia, 1977, FA Davis.
5. Gabbiani G et al: Granulation tissue as a contractile organ: a study of structure and function, *J Exp Med* 135:719–734, 1972.

6. Hubbard RP: Mechanical behavior of connective tissue. In Greenman PE, editor: *Concepts and mechanisms of neuromuscular functions,* New York, 1984, Springer-Verlag, pp 47–54.

7. Little RW: Biomechanics modeling and concepts. In Greenman PE, editor: *Concepts and mechanisms of neuromuscular functions.* New York, 1984, Springer-Verlag, pp 34–36.

8. Newham DJ et al. Pain and fatigue after eccentric and concentric muscle contractions, *Clin Sci* 64:55–62, 1983.

9. Ross R: Wound healing. *Sci Am* 220:40–50, 1969.

10. Thorstensson A, Grimby G, Karlsson J: Force-velocity relations and fiber composition in human knee extensor muscles, *J Appl Physiol* 40:12–16, 1976.

11. Wyke BD: The neurology of joints, *Ann R Coll Surg Engl* 41:25–50, 1967.

12. *International classification of impairments, disabilities and handicaps,* Geneva, Switzerland, 1980, World Health Organization.

13. Nagi SZ: Disability concepts revisited: implications to prevention. In Pope AM, Tarlov AR, editors: *Disability in America: toward a national agenda for prevention,* Washington, DC, 1991, Division of Health Promotion and Disease Prevention, Institute of Medicine. National Academic Press.

14. Fahrer H et al: Knee effusion and reflex inhibition of the quadriceps, *J Bone Joint Surg* 70:636–638.

15. Spencer JD et al: Knee joint effusion and quadriceps reflex inhibition in man, *Arch Phys Med Rehabil* 65:171–172.

TEST YOUR KNOWLEDGE

1. What is the major purpose of using a clinical decision-making model in documentation?

2. What is the classic concept that this model uses to describe orthopedic dysfunction?

3. List the four major terms for physiologic dysfunction developed by the World Health Organization (WHO), and discuss the definition of each.

4. Which one of the four WHO classifications does a physical therapist traditionally evaluate, and what tools are used to do this? What are the limitations of this approach?

5. Why is it necessary for the physical therapist to demonstrate a linkage between impairment, functional limitation, and subsequent disability?

6. What three items should be considered when determining a timeline for treatment?

7. Why is the patient's environment and previous functional level important in justifying treatment and setting treatment goals?

PRACTICE CASE STUDY

The patient, G.W., is a right-handed 53-year-old dentist who is referred to physical therapy for evaluation and treatment of a right painful, stiff shoulder.

Three months ago, while lifting a 25-hp outboard engine out of the water, the patient felt a sudden sharp pain over the anterior portion of the right shoulder, followed by burning pain over the lateral aspect of his arm (mainly in the deltoid region). When describing to you what happened, he stated that he "felt a pop." He reported that the symptoms gradually subsided over the next week, although he continued to have pain on any attempt to do overhead activities. He stopped playing tennis and working out at the health club. During the past 2 months he has noticed that he seems to be "getting stiffer" and is having difficulty working. G.W. also complains of difficulty sleeping, and is unable to lie on his right side. Finally he called a friend who is an orthopedic surgeon, who began a workup. Radiographs showed some glenohumeral joint space narrowing and mild joint effusion. There was no evidence of calcification.

G.W.'s past medical history was noncontributory, and he denies any history of a shoulder lesion. He has been taking piroxicam (Feldene). As stated earlier, G.W. is a dentist and lives with his wife and three teen-aged children.

During your examination, in addition to the above information the patient gives the following description of his problem. He complains of dull ache in the lateral aspect of his arm and in the anterior shoulder when he attempts minimal motion. His chief complaint is sharp pinching pain in the shoulder with overhead motions. He has difficulty sleeping because of the pain, and is having trouble performing routine activities of daily living. Most bothersome is the effect of the pain and inability to move his shoulder while practicing dentistry. He also indicates that he is getting very discouraged because the incessant pain is interfering with his life. He would like very much to "get rid of the pain and get back to full use of my right upper extremity." Further questioning results in denial that there is any gross weakness or neural symptoms at this time.

In further examination you note that the cervicothoracic spine radiographs are normal. On inspection you observe that there is no visible edema or effusion of the right upper extremity. The skin appears normal. However, the right shoulder is depressed and protracted, with the scapula abducted. Palpation elicits a complaint of sharp tenderness over the anterior glenohumeral joint. Further palpation reveals anterosuperior subluxation at the glenohumeral joint. There is also evidence of increased myofascial and capsular tissue density in the anterior portion of the glenohumeral joint. Further, there is a specific point of tenderness over the humeral rotator cuff insertion. Supraspinatus muscle tenderness is present throughout the supraspinatus fossa, along with marked muscle guarding of the shoulder girdle complex, particularly around the anterior deltoid, rotator cuff, upper trapezius, and pectoralis major muscles. Mild atrophy is noted in the deltoid, scapula musculature (rhomboids, middle and lower trapezius). Incidental observations reveal that the cervical spine, acromioclavicular and sternoclavicular joints, and the rest of the right upper extremity are unremarkable.

Further examination of joint mobility produces the following data. In general there is highly reactive pain felt simultaneously with anterior range of motion, posterior range of motion, and posterior range of motion with overpressure, especially in abduction and external rotation.

	Right	Left
Combined flexion	100*	170
Glenohumeral flexion	65*	90
Combined abduction	90*	180
Glenohumeral abduction	45*	90
Extension	30	60
Internal rotation	30	85
External rotation	0*	85
Elbow, hand, fingers, cervical spine	Normal	Normal

*Complaints of pain

Examination of accessory joint mobilization of the glenohumeral joint revealed the following information:

1. Distraction with + for pain and minimal excursion (grade 1)
2. Caudal glide, anteroposterior glide with + for pain and moderate excursion (grade 2)
3. Other (R/R) upper quadrant joints unremarkable for pain or mobility deficits.
4. Strength not tested at this time because of pain.

5. Neurologic manifestations unremarkable for sensory deep tendon reflex, peripheral nerve provocation tests, and myotomal deficits

Functions that specifically are bothersome are that the patient must dress the affected arm first, is unable to comb his hair using his right arm, and has abnormal gait during ambulation because he holds his right arm stiff, resulting in decreased arm swing.

Based on this case history, answer the following questions as they relate to the decision-analysis process.

1. Present a brief history of the problem.

   _____
   _____
   _____

2. Briefly detail your physical therapy examination; include comments on assessment instruments used and clinical observations.

   _____
   _____
   _____

3. Identify impairments. Support your assessment by relating it to tissue physiology and biomechanics.

4. Identify five *specific* physical therapy problems (consider tissue, structural problems, body systems, and functional problems; refer to generic goals [p 87] and Fig 3–1).

   a. _____
   b. _____
   c. _____
   d. _____
   e. _____

5. Identify *specific* short-term treatment goals for your patient. (consider specific tissue and structural goals for each problem identified in question 4).

   a. _____
      _____
   b. _____
      _____
   c. _____
      _____
   d. _____
      _____
   e. _____
      _____

6. Choose one problem from question 4 and its corresponding goal to answer the following:

   Problem: _____

   Goal: _____

   a. Describe and analyze the rationale of your goal based on tissue physiology and the mechanical behavior of contractile and/or noncontractile soft tissue. Identify *one* technique or modality, to enable you to achieve your goal: _____

   b. Describe and analyze the relationship of your technique to your goal based on tissue physiology and the mechanical behavior of contractile and/or noncontractile soft tissue.

7. Identify and discuss *three* criteria you would use to decide the magnitude, frequency, and duration of your treatment techniques for treatment session.

   a. _____

   _____

   b. _____

   _____

   _____

   c. _____

   _____

   _____

8. Relate your goal from question 6 to the Model of Orthopaedic Dysfunction by discussing how your goals relate to *three* of the following topics:

   a. Inflammation and/or tissue healing.

   _____

   _____

   b. Connective tissue—clinical behavior.

   _____

   _____

   c. Muscle structure and function.

   _____

   d. Articular neurophysiology.

   _____

   _____

   e. Cardiovascular and/or neurological implications.

   _____

   _____

   f. Soft tissue and joint biomechanics.

   _____

   _____

9. Using the clinical decision-making process further develop goals for this patient.

   Goals: _____

   _____

   _____

   _____

TEST YOUR KNOWLEDGE ANSWER SHEET

1. It provides a foundation for presentation of an appropriate treatment and documentation.

2. The model expands on the classic concept that a stimulus causes a response. It describes the sequence of events that lead to the development of limitation, disability, and handicap.

3. "Impairments" refers to the abnormalities of anatomic, physiologic, or psychologic origins within specific organs or systems of the body. "Functional limitation" refers to restrictions or inability to perform activities of daily living, such as transfers, gait, and bed mobility. "Functional disability" refers to restriction in or inability to perform a normal range of activities of daily living. "Handicap" is a much broader term. It describes limitations in the fulfillment of an individual's normal role, depending on age, sex, and other social and cultural factors.

4. Impairment. Physical therapists have traditionally focused on impairments (e.g., limitation in range of motion, muscle strength) in their evaluations. However, these impairments do not directly correlate with a patient's functional limitations or functional disabilities. For example, consider the patient, a practicing physical therapist, who has 60% reduction of right forearm pronation. This therapist has little functional limitation and *no corresponding functional disability.*

5. Linkage is necessary to form a hypothesis for dysfunction on which to build treatment interventions.

6. The three things that need to be considered when determining the time-line for treatment are the patient's response to therapy; the environment where the patient lives, works, and plays; and the patient's previous level of function.

7. The patient's environment and previous functional level are important when justifying treatment and setting goals because these factors determine the intensity of the treatment and the treatment goals. As the example, rehabilitation of an Olympic athlete requires that the therapist set a very different set of goals, adapt a different treatment approach, and provide a different intensity of treatment than for a sedentary office worker who performs no outside physical activities.

CHAPTER 4

Functional Outcome Report: The Next Generation in Physical Therapy Reporting

Gretchen Swanson, P.T., M.P.H.

Key Concepts

- Shift in reporting: a more comprehensive approach to documentation
- Evolution of reporting practices
- Functional Outcome Report: A Working Process
- Step-by-step method to functional outcome reporting
- Subsequent functional outcome reports: sustained performance model

SHIFT IN REPORTING: A MORE COMPREHENSIVE APPROACH TO DOCUMENTATION

The decade of the 1980s was a watershed era for the physical therapy profession. Never before were opportunities for the autonomy and professional advancement of physical therapists so great. It was also a time of increasing pressure from consumers and payers to insist that therapists prove they can produce and document the results of the services they provide. The decade of the 1990s is shaped by the **Americans With Disabilities Act** (ADA) of 1990 (*Federal Register*, July 26, 1991). This landmark legislation forces the distinction between impairment and disability. Physical therapists will increasingly be asked to define functional limitations, particularly at the job site, and to recommend methods to improve, eliminate, or accommodate residual disability. This important shift in the responsibilities of the physical therapist, as well as the expectations of consumers and payers who receive and pay for therapy services, has led to some equally important changes in reporting requirements.

Reporting for physical therapy services now requires analysis of the functional consequences of the medical condition or disease and the functional result of the physical therapy provided. Because the focus of the physical therapy report has changed, the format of the report needs to change as well. Hence, in reporting models proposed today you will encounter a great number of terms, such as **impairment, movement dysfunction, disability, activity restriction,** function, and **outcome.** These terms, and the important concepts they represent, influence the type of physical therapy report you write.

In new reporting requirements, it is no longer acceptable to report that the patient's symptoms have improved. It is now expected that a report describe the functional consequence of the symptoms and that there is a linkage between the function and meaningful activities. For example, if a patient came to physical therapy complaining of leg pain and your report indicated that treatment had relieved the pain, previously that would have been considered a positive treatment outcome. Today you also need to include functional consequences. Using the previous example, a functional consequence could be that the patient *achieved the ability to tolerate driving a car for at least 1 hour,* an activity the patient had been unable to accomplish because of the symptom of pain.

This chapter introduces the concepts of functional outcome reporting. We explore how to apply these concepts to daily practice and discuss how you can use a Functional Outcome Report (FOR) system[1] to improve the way you deliver services to patients. We also explore examples of documentation that clearly demonstrate functional consequences of treatment intervention. We discuss three aspects of outcome associated with a FOR system, which by definition must demonstrate meaningful, practical, and sustainable outcomes. Through sample reports you will learn how to extend documentation beyond the traditional problem-oriented reporting model based on impairment to include functional outcome considerations. Learning these concepts will influence how you shape your practice and referral patterns and enhance your status as a professional services provider in a managed care environment.

EVOLUTION OF REPORTING PRACTICES

SOAP: Fallacies of Simplistic Goal-setting

Most physical therapists who were educated before the 1980s, many of whom are in practice today, were taught to chart daily physical therapy sessions according to **SOAP** (subjective, objective, assessment, and plan), a component of the **Problem-Oriented Medical Record** (POMR).[1] Summary SOAP notes (Table 4–1) were traditionally considered good record-keeping.[2,3] Therapists were trained to believe that recording a patient's report of "less pain" or the therapist's observations of "increased strength" constituted satisfactory charting and, by extension, quality care.

The SOAP format was certainly easy to use, and satisfied the documentation requirements of the period. SOAP notes allowed the physical therapist to quickly record the patient's complaint, the therapist's objective findings, and whether any change in symptoms or physical findings occurred.

This style of reporting contains a built-in bias because it assumes that improvement in physical capabilities leads directly to improved function. This is not always the case. In the SOAP example, we can assume that increasing the patient's lower extremity strength will lead to improved standing function and that therefore no further analysis or justification for treatment is needed. In reality, in many types of disorders an increase in lower body strength alone will not result in the patient's ability to stand. Because the SOAP style of reporting does not control for this bias, it is not sufficient to demonstrate that the treatment plan is appropriate. To avoid this bias and assure that appropriate and accountable care is provided, amore structured approach to reporting functional assessment and outcome is needed.

TABLE 4–1.

BRIEF SOAP NOTE

Subjective: "I feel better today, not so much pain on the right side. I'm beginning to stand for short periods of time."

Objective: Patient with muscle tightness pre-stretching of hamstrings, now with 50% range of movement of low back/hip flexion in long sitting. Performs exercises correctly.

Assessment: Patient unable to stand longer than 5 minutes without complaint of pain responds to soft tissue techniques and use of ultrasound for up to 3 hours. Since start of care 2 weeks ago for low back strain, patient has improved.

Plan: Continue physical therapy treatment.

Need for Better System

In the 1980s two important changes occurred in the practice of physical therapy: therapists became more autonomous, and a better method of documenting outcomes became a clear-cut necessity.[4-8]

The physical therapy profession became more sophisticated. Physical therapy professionals began to place greater emphasis on research, clinical theories, and diagnostic definitions and classifications. At the same time, better educational opportunities and stricter requirements emerged for those seeking career advancement through clinical specialization, advanced degrees, and postgraduate residencies. More recently, increased interest in greater mastery of orthopedics, neurology, and numerous other clinical areas has generated a range of intensive workshops, some leading to specialization.

As greater physical therapy competency emerged, there was an unrelated but coincident nationwide increase in expenditure for physical therapy services. As the costs of services began to rise dramatically throughout the United States, third-party payers began to insist that physical therapists, through reporting, justify why therapy was necessary.[9-14] This new requirement was in sharp contrast to earlier expectations, in which it was assumed that if the patient had a physical limitation, that in itself was sufficient justification for treatment.

For the first time, physical therapists were being challenged to account for the services they provided. Their responses were understandably confusing and voluminous. They were faced with time-consuming paperwork and few guidelines for satisfying these new reporting requests. Their handwritten reports were often packed with acronyms, abbreviations, and clipped sentences in an attempt to record more and more detail and to include additional test findings (Table 4–2). In response, payers escalated their requests for in-depth reports at a rate that continued to reflect the nationwide increases in expenditures for physical therapy.[15-19]

One possible benefit of these changes in reporting requirements was that physical therapists became better observers and recorders of the results of their services. However, it soon became evident to physical therapists and payers alike that simply expanding the existing system of note taking was not working. The *quality*, not just the *quantity*, of reporting needed to change.

In recent years, cost escalation and resources available for health care have exceeded payers' ability to continue to pay for unlimited services. As a result, payers have had to develop medically based criteria for use in payment decisions in order to meet the needs of the consumer and to meet the

TABLE 4–2.

EXPANDED **SOAP** NOTE

Diagnosis: Status post right shoulder replacement with denervation of deltoid; electromyographic evidence of reinnervation.

Treatment Request: Shoulder rehabilitation.

History: Patient is well-known to this therapist. Returns for continuation of therapy after a fall sustained 5 months ago, at which time physician deferred physical therapy treatment.

Initial Evaluation

Strength (manual muscle test)

Right anterior deltoid: 2+/5
Right middle deltoid: 2+/5
Right posterior deltoid: 3−/5

Active/passive range of motion

Right shoulder flexion: 30/180 degrees
Right shoulder abduction: 90/180 degrees
Right shoulder external: rotation: 45/50 degrees
Right shoulder internal rotation: 90/90 degrees

Electrical stimulation: right deltoid

DC current: Uncomfortable; brisk muscle contraction
AC current: Comfortable; some muscle fiber contraction (at level 3 intensity)

Treatment of supervised therapeutic exercise: right shoulder

1. Abduction: supine with skate and 3-lb weight
2. Extention-rotation: supine without weight
3. Flexion: sidelying on left without weight
4. Elbow extensors: sitting with 3-lb weight
5. Elbow flexors: sitting with 4-lb weight

Assessment: Reinnervation occurring. Tolerates treatment well.

Plan: Continue with therapeutic exercise to increase muscle strength to grade 3. Reinitiate pool for weightless exercise to right upper extremity and continue electrical stimulation with DC or AC current, depending on patient comfort level. Combined program to occur three times per week for 8 weeks.

demands of the public. There no longer are endless resources for financing medical and rehabilitation care. Dollar limits for specific services are being set to protect the resources of both patient and payer. In relation to physical therapy services, this means that *functional outcome* is the key to justification of services and successful reimbursement. Therefore the documentation method must be structured on functional outcome so that the therapist and others can successfully track and record outcomes.

To be considered a functional outcome, the activity, by definition, must be:

1. *Meaningful* to the patient and/or caregiver. The ability achieved by the patient through physical therapy is necessary for the patient to function most effectively at home or at work.
2. *Practical to the patient.* The most economical and efficient means are used to assist the patient to achieve the desired ability.
3. *Sustainable over time.* The level of function achieved during the course of physical therapy is maintained by the patient outside of the clinical environment over time.

There has not been a universally accepted model for functional outcome reporting. Any such system should be a comprehensive, flexible process that benefits the physical therapist, the payer, and the patient alike. It should be an ongoing process that develops in relation to the patient's changing functional activities. The model presented in this chapter was developed by Swanson,[1] and is used to illustrate one approach. Regardless of the model used, it should include the following concepts:

1. It should rely on observable, testable patient function over time.
2. It should relate to any therapy model or setting.
3. It should allow the physical therapist to apply *clinical reasoning* to determine both the underlying cause and functional consequence of the disorder.
4. It should distinguish the concepts of diagnosis and impairment from the functional consequence of the disorder.
5. It should permit more accurate, useful prediction of outcomes, necessary in a cost-containment and managed care health care system.
6. It should provide patients and therapists with more realistic, meaningful objectives.
7. It should provide a rationale for requesting payment of services during the necessary course of physical therapy care.

FUNCTIONAL OUTCOME REPORT: A WORKING PROCESS

The functional outcome report (FOR) meets the aforementioned criteria because it is a comprehensive and specific method of translating clinical reasoning into a report that will satisfy payer requirements, lead to more effective monitoring of patient performance, and more than meet ADA guidelines. Within this structure, functional outcome is not seen as an existing list of functions and cannot be constructed in the abstract. It is, in a concrete sense, a specific set of behaviors, tasks, or activities required for a particular patient to achieve optimum functional levels outside the clinical environment.

Within this model, the functional outcome is always determined in light of the patient's medical condition and is monitored throughout the period of care. The reporting system is a six-step system (Table 4–3).

The system relies on functional activities that meet the three critical criteria of being meaningful, practical, and sustainable over time.[20] With these three criteria in mind, let us explore how the FOR system works in daily practice.

From Clinical Reasoning to Reporting Functional Outcomes

It is important to understand that reporting forms and formats are not and cannot be substitutes for completion of a thorough clinical reasoning process such as the orthopedic model presented in Chapter 3. Another model, which presents a neurologic dysfunction approach, is presented in Appendix II–B. The FOR differs from other documentation approaches that purport that "If you will only do these things" or "If you will only fill in these blanks" your reporting will improve.

In the past, physical therapists analyzed treatment based on a medical impairment model, which included assessment of the cause, the disease or injury, and the patients resultant physical status. This model assumed that if the patient's physical status improved (e.g., strength increased) there would be concomitant improvement in the patient's ability to function, such as the ability to walk. There is no scientific basis for this assumption.[21, 22] More important, physical therapists are being challenged with increasing fre-

TABLE 4–3.

SIX STEPS IN FUNCTIONAL OUTCOME REPORT MODEL BY SWANSON (FOR)

Step	Clinical Reasoning Process	FOR Report Item
1	Establish patient needs	Report reason for referral
2	Analyze patient performance	Identify and report functional limitation
3	Identify clinician impression	Establish physical therapy assessment
4	Postulate relationships between impairment and performance	Identify therapy problems
5	Predict functional outcome	List functional outcome goals
6	Devise treatment strategy	Present treatment plan and rationale

quency to demonstrate that the treatment has a significant effect on the patient's functional outcome that would not have occurred otherwise.[23-26]

STEP-BY-STEP METHOD TO FUNCTIONAL OUTCOME REPORTING

Your reporting role as a physical therapist is to document the functional consequences of a disorder. The FOR method relies on the therapist's expertise to gather information, assess the patient's physical therapy needs, and plan an effective treatment program. It also operates from a clinical analysis perspective, which requires the therapist to use sound clinical reasoning to present an appropriate and acceptable rationale for treatment. The rationale serves as a basis for reporting *meaningful, practical, and sustainable outcomes.* In doing so, the report should describe how the physical limitations or impairments caused by the patient's medical condition have an impact on the patient's ability to execute specific tasks or perform desired activities, usually activities needed to live or work outside the clinical environment. The steps of FOR guide the therapist through the reporting process. It not only includes testing impairment or observation of movement dysfunction, but also proceeds through a process of describing the functional consequence or loss, for example, *limitation in community ambulation, inability to lift packages heavier than 50 pounds, or cannot drive a car* safely.

The definitions within the FOR system are derived from a number of therapy scholars and clinicians. Most important is the work of Sahrmann, and then Rose, in developing the conceptual framework of a physical therapy assessment and diagnosis. Jette[7, 29] has underscored the need for functionally based reports, and Swanson[5, 6] has defined the need for skilled physical therapy, therapy problems and outcomes management. Finally, the concept of *reason for referral* comes from Allen and Earhart,[27] occupational therapy scholars noted for development of request-for-services analysis prior to admission for therapy services.

Table 4–4 illustrates how the clinical reasoning process (see orthopedic model in Chapter 3) also leads to the step-by-step FOR documentation process. Table 4–5 is a sample functional outcome report form, and Table 4–6 is an example of a completed initial functional outcome report. Based on these examples, we will examine each stage of the FOR process, that is,

1. How each step in clinical reasoning leads to each entry of an initial functional outcome report.
2. How to complete a subsequent report to maintain the FOR system for your patients.

TABLE 4-4.

USE OF CLINICAL REASONING TO CREATE FUNCTIONAL OUTCOME REPORT

Step	Clinical Decision Model	Clinical Reasoning Process	FOR Report Item
1	History of present problem	Establish *patient* need based on *patient*/caregiver *complaint*	Reason for referral
2	Initial physical therapy examination	*Analyze performance* based on test findings and clinical observation	Functional limitations (including activity restrictions)
3	Identify impairment; report results (PT diagnosis: identify altered physical state causing activity restriction and/or physical impairment causing movement dysfunction)	Identify *Clinical impression*	Physical therapy assessment Elaborate on medical diagnosis and report positive test findings, impairments, movement dysfunction
4	Initial problem list	Postulate *relationships* between *impairments* and *performance* based on medical condition, PT assessment, patient performance	Therapy problems
5	Set treatment goals	*Predict functional outcome,* based on therapist judgment and expertise	Functional outcome goals
6	Select specific techniques	Devise *treatment* strategy	Treatment plan and rationale

Step 1—Establishing Patient Needs: Reporting Reason for Referral

Patients typically come to physical therapy with a specific physical complaint. The physical complaint by the patient is another way to describe what the patient needs to achieve as a result of the course of physical therapy care. All too frequently assumptions are made by both the patient and the therapist as to the patient's functional concerns. In the FOR and other systems, the physical therapist needs to investigate the complaint thoroughly before proceeding with the examination or developing a treatment strategy. *Unless an analysis in terms of need and priority to the patient is made, the therapist will find it difficult to determine when the goals have been achieved.*

One way to assure that this analysis occurs is to use a systematic and routine set of interview questions, which helps to establish the basis for the FOR. Allen and Earhart[27] have developed an effective way in which to uniformly evaluate the patient's needs (Appendix II–D).

TABLE 4–5.

SAMPLE FUNCTIONAL OUTCOME REPORT FORM

Reason for referral		
Functional Limitations		
Activity	*Current Performance Status*	
PT assessment		
Therapy problems		
Functional outcome goals		
Activity	*Target Performance Status*	*Due Date*
Treatment plan with Rationale		

It is important to remember that the first criteria of a functional outcome is that it be meaningful to the patient or caregiver. It is not unusual after a course of physical therapy for patients to have **residual impairments** (e.g., reduced joint motion or muscle strength) and **residual disabilities** (e.g., require a walker to ambulate about the home or a job site modification to ac-

TABLE 4–6.

INITIAL FUNCTIONAL OUTCOME REPORT

Reason for Referral

Patient post meniscectomy of left knee reports pain, stiffness, and difficulty with walking and other upright mobility activities

Functional limitations

Activity	Current Status
Sit-to-stand transfer	Independent
Standing balance	Performs independently, with cane
Flat terrain ambulation (speed)	
Flat terrain ambulation (endurance)	Performs with cane for more than 18 sec for 20 ft
	Tolerates less than 5 min
Ambulation on uneven terrain	Unable
Stair climbing	Ascends two steps, descends two steps with railing and minimum assistance

PT assessment

Medical diagnosis status post meniscectomy is further defined to include residual left knee joint inflammation

Positive test findings: Positive fluctuation test; limited strength; quadriceps 3/5 and hamstrings 4/5, indicative of synovial effusion

Therapy problems

1. Pain on compression maneuvers of the left knee: sitting, sit to stance, periodically during gait cycle, during all phases of stair climbing
2. Difficulty in coordinating gait cycle with use of cane to reduce stress to left knee

Functional outcome goals

Activity	Performance	Due date
Flat terrain ambulation (speed)	Independent without device; 20 ft in 9 s	Within 14 days
Flat terrain ambulation (endurance)	Tolerates unassisted walking for 30 min	Within 21 days
Uneven terrain ambulation	Tolerates for a minimum of 15 min	Within 14 days
Stair climbing	Ascends and descends 15 steps	Within 21 days

Treatment plan with rationale

Application of anti-inflammatory modalities with instruction for follow-up home program to minimize post-activity edema

Lower extremity strength training with instruction in progressive home exercise program

Patient instructed in activity limits and restrictions during the course of care.

commodate materials handling limitation), yet achieve meaningful functional outcomes.

In the case of a patient returning to work, careful review of the patient's essential job functions will assist in identifying tasks, elements of tasks, and composite activities needed to fulfill job requirements. For example after several flare-up episodes of rheumatoid arthritis, a patient has reduction of motion in both hands. Through the interview process the patient states that both driving and home activities are hampered, and that driving is an essential function of his job. If return to work is the basis for the referral, the therapist is being requested to improve the patient's capacity to drive. Although this patient has a residual impairment, he is capable of achieving independence in a functional area of importance to him.

Once the patient's complaint or functional concern is thoroughly investigated, it should be entered on the initial report under "Reason for referral." This statement should also reflect the physical change that has caused the patient to lose physical function, and indicate factors that have led to restriction of activities (see Tables 4–4 and 4–5). The decreased ability to perform particular functions should not be viewed in isolation, but should be considered as a functional consequence of the patient's disease or injury (e.g., the medical diagnosis). This decrease in ability to function becomes the baseline for determining the patient's therapy goal during the period of physical therapy.

Step 2—Analyzing Patient Performance: Identifying and Reporting Functional Limitations

After noting the reason for referral, the therapist should next test and observe the patient in order to draw conclusions as to the specific cause of the complaint. To clearly understand this step in the FOR process, a discussion of functional assessment is helpful. It is important to clearly recognize what functional tests are and what they are not, and how to report loss of function in a FOR.

Functional Assessment
Functional assessment means exactly what it says: assessment of the function, or set of purposeful actions, an individual is expected to perform under optimum conditions. Because the word functional implies so much to physical therapists, a classification of purposeful actions is used here to illustrate the variety of functions that pertain to physical therapy.

Purposeful Action	Examples
Elements of tasks	Reaching, stepping, sit-to-stand
Specific tasks	Lower body dressing, flat terrain ambulation
Composite activities	Driving, shopping, working at a desk

Although there may be a variety of purposeful actions that the patient wants to achieve as a result of physical therapy, the most important step is to select the tasks or activities that will serve as measures and predictors of a successful physical therapy outcome. Remember to choose the task and activities that are:

- Most valuable (meaningful) to the patient and/or caregiver
- Most applicable (practical) to this episode of physical therapy
- Most treatable (sustainable) by physical therapy procedures

If you select an element of a task, you need to consider the tasks or composite activity in which it will be used. You may choose to evaluate and monitor a single task, such as room ambulation. This task may include the components of walking within a familiar room containing objects that can be used for support, allowing the patient to become more self-sufficient at home. This task is not the same as walking on a city street. Therefore, simply reporting the patient's ability to ambulate fails to adequately describe the patient's function.

Functional Assessment Tests

In many cases, you may need to evaluate and monitor a number of functions for a particular patient. If this is the case, you may wish to consider using a functional assessment test. These tests have become the focus of some controversy in recent years.[28] Questions have been raised as to whether they are valid, reliable, or meaningful. Some of the questions raised[31-36] regarding functional assessment tests include the following:

1. Does the test assess *capacity* or *performance, capability* or *disability*? That is, *could* the patient perform the task or *does* the patient *perform* the task? Are you asking what *can* the patient do or what *can't* the patient do? More often than not, patients want to know if they *could do* it, and you and the payer want to know if they *do* it.

2. Does the test control for devices or for motivation? There is an important distinction between internal (motivational) and external (environmental) controls. Does the test allow you to differentiate whether additional controls are used, and if so, were they required in order for the patient to complete the task? It is not unusual for a patient to perform quite satisfactorily in the clinical setting, where the heights of objects, minimum distraction, assistance from staff, and other factors all serve to improve the patient's performance. However, when the patient's spouse or caregiver attempts to carry out the same activity with the patient in the home environment, the patient fails to perform at the same level.

3. What is the effect of the rater on the score? This is undoubtedly one of physical therapy's biggest measurement dilemmas. To complete an accurate FOR, you must be convinced that your score reliably reflects the patient's performance. Therefore, your observation, testing, or interview methodology must be rigorous.

4. How meaningful is a generic inventory of activities to all patients? In some circumstances (e.g., screening mobility skills in a nursing home) an inventory of activities may prove an easy and economic way to select pa-

tients who need further physical therapy services. But unless there is a situation in which all patients you treat require the same minimal functional level, a generic inventory will not be useful in your FOR.

5. Are you assessing level of care (e.g., for a patient who needs supervision in all activities) or level of performance (e.g., the ability to lift 10-lb boxes at hourly intervals on the job)? The difference demands use of different rating scales, such as, minimum, moderate, or maximum assistance, vs. a rating scale that precisely indicates parameters of the completed task, such as weight, distance, and speed.

6. Can the functional test be used repeatedly to obtain valid results?

A plethora of literature is available regarding the validity of functional tests, and you are encouraged to review it. When selecting a test you should decide which of these questions are important to you and your patients in preparing the report. Once this has been established, it is possible to locate or create a functional assessment tool appropriate to your setting. One sample tool, the "Western Physical Performance Analysis" (WPPA),[37]* is found in Appendix II–C. The WPPA is a functional assessment tool designed for the severely disabled head injured population.

If you already have access to a functional test that answers all of these questions to your satisfaction, you may be well-advised to use it. Because no universal tool is available to physical therapists to test function, most compile a small library of useful ones. In the final analysis, the best guide to follow in deciding to use an assessment test is whether it meets the criteria of testing for meaningful, practical, and sustainable functional outcomes.[38–40]

What Functional Assessment Testing is Not

Functional assessment testing is not simply a number of rated physical performance tasks. A trip to a physical therapy conference exhibit hall will quickly update you on a number of so-called "functional assessment systems." Most of these testing methodologies are essentially ways to uniformly test and re-test single tasks or activities. Some of these tests are informative to the clinician and occasionally to the patient. As a group, however, they typically fail to address the needs of the patient, caregiver, employer, and payer. Ultimately it is up to the physical therapist to interpret the patient's performance on a test battery, taking all the clinical findings and the patient's needs into account.

---

*Available from Director of Therapy Services, Western Neuro Care, PO Box 170, Tustin, CA 92681-0170.

Reporting Functional Limitations

The initial interview will have provided you with a list of functional tasks and activities relevant to the patient. For example, your interview findings show that the patient is unable to perform some essential job functions adequately. Of particular importance to your patient may be the ability to lift, as this hampers all other aspects of the job. You have evaluated your patient's lifting performance with certain indicators in mind, such as lifting a 10- to 15-lb box from a waist-high surface. The patient's performance of purposeful actions must be rated and documented.

The parameters of rating of such actions most often used are as follows:

1. *Tolerance.* Can the task be completed once? Are assistive devices, environmental adaptations, or other reasonable accommodations available and appropriate, or is physical assistance required to complete the task?

2. *Endurance.* Can the task be repeated? How often can it be repeated within a given time period?

3. *Performance response.* Is the speed and accuracy at the desired levels? Does performing the task increase pain, fatigue, or limit the patient's ability to perform other tasks? Does the performance deteriorate over time?

The rating scales to describe each of these parameters depends on what is considered normal or desirable for the patient. In the example above, lifting can be measured in terms of lifts per minute or per hour. It also is the objective scale to monitor your patient's achieved outcome.

The result of the ratings of such actions lead to a statement of functional limitations. When formulating such statements, the physical therapy community frequently interchanges the terms **activity restriction, functional limitation,** and **disability.** Each of these terms suggest that the individual's function has been negatively affected by the underlying physical disorder. Although any one of these terms may be applied to a given case,[41–43] it is important to understand how they are interpreted by different types of payers. For example, if you were reporting to Medicare, you might use the term disability to describe a patient's inability to ambulate in the community as a functional consequence of a neurological dysfunction. In the Workers Compensation system, only a physician can make the determination of disability or the inability to return to work. Therefore, when submitting a report to a physician in a Worker's Compensation case, you would use either activity restriction or functional limitation to describe the patient's inability to ambulate on uneven terrain as a functional consequence of a work-related injury.

To avoid these inconsistencies in interpretation, and meet the spirit of the Americans With Disabilites Act, a better more meaningful approach is to report your findings in functional terms. The functional consequence of any given physical disorder can usually be described as an activity restriction of one kind or another. When reporting the patient's activity restriction, you are defining the patient's functional limitations in terms of the specific tasks and actions that the individual is expected to perform with an optimal therapeutic outcome. This reasoning process of defining activity restriction will not only assist you in reporting the patient's functional limitations, it will also help to establish *meaningful, practical,* and *sustainable* goals for the patient as time goes on.

The activity restrictions you report are based on patient and caregiver needs as well as on your observations and test ratings of the patient's current performance levels. Under "Functional Limitations," on the report form, list each specific task or activity tested and your analysis of the patient's ability to perform each one. The list of activity restrictions must identify the specific task or activity, the severity of the limitation, and the degree of assistance needed, if any. In relation to the purposeful actions described earlier, the types of activity restrictions frequently reported by physical therapists are those shown on page 112.

Step 3—Identifying Clinician Impression: Physical Therapy Assessment

Once you have completed the performance analysis and have identified the functional limitations, you are ready to formulate a **physical therapy assessment.** Whether you use the term physical therapy assessment or physical therapy diagnosis, the definition as it applies in this discussion is "the identification of the altered physical status that has caused the activity restriction." This assessment is different from the medical diagnosis in that it focuses on the functional consequences of the disease or disorder rather than simply the precipitating cause. It specifically addresses the physical impairment that has caused the movement or mobility component of the functional deficit.

Physical therapy assessments describe physical impairments, such as alterations in contractile tissue, changes in articular structure, sensory changes, and movement dysfunctions (reduction in strength or muscle tone, or loss of motor control). When reporting, the therapist should write the assessment as though it were an extension or elaboration of the medical diagnosis.

The term **impairment** has received a great deal of attention since the International Classification of Impairments, Disabilities, and Handicaps

(ICIDH), published in 1980.[42] A discussion of these issues as they relate to physical therapy is included for your information.

How ICIDH Classification System Relates To Physical Therapy Reporting

The International Classification of Impairments, Disabilities, and Handicaps (ICIDH) system* has proved useful to policy makers who need a uniform, easily understood method within which to interpret the need for ongoing rehabilitation services.[42] Like the *ICD-9* codes used universally for medical diagnosis, the ICIDH codes represent a potential method for reporting functional outcomes.

However, the ICIDH system of categorizing the consequences of disease and injury remains problematic for physical therapists. The major problems with the current system are (1) the inadequacy of terms used to describe impairment; (2) omission of a physical therapy assessment within its conceptual framework; and (3) the use of the label "disability," rather than "activity restriction" or "functional limitation," to describe the functional consequence of a disorder.

Clinical application of the ICIDH codes continues to be limited as a result of the terms chosen for impairments (e.g., longitudinal deficiency of the radius or mechanical impairment of the ankle and foot). A sample of ICIDH codes are found in Appendix II–A. Many of the terms used are unfamiliar to physical therapists in the United States. More important, these impairment designations do little to interpret the physical alterations relative to the restricted activity it causes and the therapy that might treat it.

These problems with the ICIDH have, in fact, challenged a number of authors and scientists to offer alternative definitions and solutions. Guccione[43] and Jette,[44] in separate articles, have discussed the concept of functional limitation relative to the ICIDH system. Nagi[45] has proposed a system that includes functional limitation but does not offer terms, labels, or codes for clinical reporting purposes.

Basis for the Functional Outcome Report

Impairments may indicate damage to a single anatomic structure or physiologic function, or reduced effect of a confluence of multiple systems.[46, 47] Therefore, each impairment influences the patient's function and treatment strategy in a different way. In contrast to the **medical impairment model** used with the SOAP reporting format, the clinical reasoning process reflected in the functional outcome reporting system addresses a model based

---

*Available from WHO Publications Centre USA, 49 Sheridan Ave., Albany, NY 12210.

on the influence of the impairment on function. This approach relates to the patient's physical impairment-movement disorder-activity restriction as an interactive set of factors. These factors are illustrated in Table 4–7 and Figure 4–1.

A functional outcome reasoning process requires that the therapist logically identify the activity, in addition to the underlying injury or pathology, as part of the problem. These factors will influence how the therapist evaluates and treats the given activity restriction. An example of a neurologic dysfunction model is found in Appendix II–B.

Step 4—Postulating Relationships Between Impairments and Performance, Leading to Identification of Therapy Problems

The next step is the identification of therapy problems that assist in defining the elements of the altered physical status. It identifies *which of the elements will be changed as a result of physical therapy or, once changed, will improve the patient's functional status*. Examples of therapy problems include inadequate balance response during standing transfers, incomplete gleno-humeral motion during reaching, and pain as a result of prolonged flexed position (such as sitting).

The FOR approach guides the therapist to translate therapy problems to the reviewer audience using a three-step drill:

1. Description of impairment or movement dysfunction
2. Measurement used, and test findings
3. Relationship to the patient's loss in function or activity restriction

This translation helps the reader understand why physical therapy is needed and makes understandable the treatment that is subsequently recommended. A few sample translations are shown in Table 4–8. For example, in many

TABLE 4–7.

COMPARISON OF MEDICAL IMPAIRMENT AND FUNCTIONAL OUTCOME MODELS

Factor	Medical Impairment Model	Functional Outcome Model
Tests	Physical findings/impairments	Physical findings/impairments (in relationship to pathology)
	Residual disability	Activity restrictions (and probable residual disability)
Assessment	Disease/disorder	Movement dysfunction (as a result of impairment)
Outcome	Reduction in signs, symptoms, and impairment	Reduction in disability

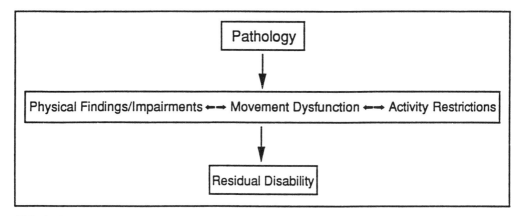

FIG 4–1.
Basis of physical therapy assessment and Functional Outcome Report.

geriatric settings, both patient and caregiver need to have an assessment of the patient's current safety status during transfers and home ambulation in order to determine the patient's potential for independent status and/or improvement after illness or injury. The physical therapist must compare clinical findings such as muscle strength, coordination, balance, and cognition with the patient's baseline function *in a specific task* to assess whether improvement is possible. Successive monitoring of the patient's functional status in the activity will verify whether the therapist's prediction was correct.

TABLE 4–8.

Examples of Translations of Therapy Problems

Impairment/Movement Dysfunction	Measurement/Findings	Relationship to Function
Left lower extremity weakness	Manual muscle test Left quadriceps 2/5 Left hamstrings 3/5	Left knee buckles on heel strike; patient speed and safety in gait compromised
Restricted head and neck movement	Swallow flouroscopy; incomplete swallow	Patient at risk for aspiration pneumonia
Incoordination in both upper extremities	Behavioral task analysis Time exceeds limits for normal elderly	Patient unable to complete hair combing, clothes donning, toothbrushing, without continuous guidance and within tolerable timeframe for caregiver.
Temperomandibular joint dysfunction	Positive Chvostek test	Limited bite and chewing; patient unable to consume full meals without food alteration

Step 5—Predicting a Functional Outcome: Functional Outcome Goals

For years, therapists have been asked to establish short-term and long-term goals. Attempts were made in the early 1980s to encourage therapists to use measurable statements, such as "Patient will increase ambulation to 40 ft." All too frequently, these statements were never referred to again in subsequent reports. As in the first two examples of SOAP notes (see Tables 4–1 and 4–2), little consideration was given to the effect, consequence, or outcome that physical therapy might have in addressing the physical disorder.

The three key factors in setting meaningful, practical, and sustainable goals are function, outcome, and prediction. As a physical therapist, your responsibility to your patients is to predict the functional outcome of treatment. It assures continuity of care, especially when ongoing or extended care is needed.

Many physical therapists are uncomfortable with the idea of prediction. However, prediction is the only useful tool for goal setting. It serves to justify your services to the patient and/or caregiver, as well as to the payer. If you are unsure of your ability to predict your patient's outcomes, ask yourself the following question. *If you do not know what the effect of your treatment will be, who does? If you cannot predict the outcome of your therapeutic services, why should your patients expose themselves to it?*

In reporting functional outcome goals, I suggest using the following format (see Table 4–6) to assure that your predictions are credible.

1. *Function.* State the activities or tasks that are most meaningful to the patient and/or caregiver.
2. *Predict outcome.* Describe the level of physical assistance, or severity of limitation and/or task modification, for each function that the patient will achieve at the end of this course of therapy care. *Short-term goals* are considered to be what the patient will achieve at the end of the current billing period, referral period, or other meaningful interval. *Long-term goals* are what will ultimately be achieved by the patient at the time of discharge.

Step 6—Devising a Treatment Strategy: Treatment Plan With Rationale

Using established theory and study findings, along with your own predictions based on clinical reasoning as discussed, you are ready to explore therapeutic alternatives for the patient and to decide on a treatment plan. The treatment plan is written to inform both the patient and the reader of the report about how the treatment will directly alter the patient's physical status and the functional consequences of that patient's disorder. For example, the therapist's report states that a patient's pain status is related to prolonged inflammation (physical therapy assessment) and results in an antalgic gait pattern (therapy problem), then a treatment strategy that counters the cause (e.g., use of an anti-inflammatory agent such as ice; limited weight bearing) would be a reasonable treatment plan.

SUBSEQUENT FUNCTIONAL OUTCOME REPORTS: SUSTAINED-PERFORMANCE MODEL

Once the initial FOR process has been completed, it will be easy for the physical therapist to develop subsequent reports that demonstrate the validity and effectiveness of the predicted outcome. Tables 4–9 and 4–10 illustrate these concepts.

The key to subsequent FORs is to report sustained change during the course of your physical therapy care. Frequently therapists use what is referred to as a "test-retest" approach, in which the therapist rates performance initially. Over the course of care, the therapist continues to retest and to report any changes that occur as a result of the treatment. Common test parameters used to indicate change include change in speed, accuracy, and endurance within a functional activity. For example, the patient requires the maximum assistance of two people for room ambulation once a day following surgery, and after 4 weeks of therapy is able to ambulate in the room with a walker and with minimum assistance from one person during all self-care activities.

The requirement for documenting test–re-test findings is not new and continues to be requested by referrers and payers of physical therapy services. The FOR model is unique. It differs from the traditional before-after method in that it does not rely exclusively on the initial level of function

TABLE 4–9.

Using Clinical Reasoning to Create a Subsequent Functional Outcome Report

Record of Clinical Action	Chart Item
Observation of movement dysfunction	Daily note
Retest impairments	Daily note
Monitor performance within specific activities	Daily and weekly notes
Verify functional outcome prediction	Subsequent FOR (progress note)

TABLE 4–10.

SUBSEQUENT FUNCTIONAL OUTCOME REPORT (AFTER THREE TREATMENT SESSIONS)

Physical therapy assessment
Residual knee joint inflammation. Positive test findings at the time of initial evaluation include positive fluctuation test, indicating significant synovial effusion

Current therapy problems
1. Pain reduced on compression maneuvers of the left knee: limited to prolonged sitting and repeated stair climbing
2. Difficulty in coordinating gait cycle with use of cane has been eliminated; the only problem that remains is the need to limit the patient's activity

Functional limitations

Activity	Initial status	Current status
Sit-to-stand transfer	Independent	Performs independently
Standing balance	Performs independently with cane	with or without cane
Flat terrain ambulation (speed)	Performs with cane for more than 18 sec for 20 ft	Performs with cane for 13.5 sec for 20 ft
Flat terrain ambulation (endurance)	Tolerates less than 5 min	Tolerates 10 min
Uneven terrain ambulation	Unable	Unable
Stair climbing	Ascends two steps, descends two steps with railing and minimum assistance	Ascends/descends with cane independently

Functional outcome goals

Activity	Target performance level	Due date
Ambulation, flat terrain		
Speed	Independent without device 20 ft in 9 sec	10 days
Endurance	Tolerates 30 min of unassisted walking	15 days
Ambulation, uneven terrain		
Endurance	Tolerates minimum of 15 steps	10 days
Stair climbing	Ascends/descends 15 steps	21 days

Treatment plan, with rationale
Patient has progressed with all mobility skills. There is a marked reduction of pain with left knee compression during testing and mobility tasks. Limited physical therapy intervention is need to eliminate residual joint inflammation and limit patient's activity level until there are no residual signs of synovial effusion.

Advance lower extremity strength training with instruction in progressive home exercise program, to include greater duration and resistance. Patient is to continue with anti-inflammatory, edema management program at home. Patient to be reinstructed in activity limits and restrictions during the course of care, including signs and symptoms of overexertion and prolonged activity duration.

and a single re-test to determine outcome, but also relies on the critical concept of **sustained performance** to demonstrate that change has occurred. Ottenbacher[49] describes the test–re-test method for therapy services in an interesting and easy-to-read manner, and his book may be a valuable resource for your professional library. Familiarity with recent applications of motor learning theory to documentation of sustained change in function as a result of physical therapy intervention may also be helpful. Valid testing and subsequent reporting of changes in motor performance require an understanding of these theories. These theories are thoroughly addressed in a recent series of articles on movement science,[50] particularly an article by Winstein.[51] Motor learning approaches, as an adjunct to validation of improved performance, apply not only to the neurologically impaired patient but also to orthopedic and cardiopulmonary impaired patients.

When addressing the issues of validity in testing of performance, testing must demonstrate that the patient has learned new movement behavior and therefore has advanced or improved in function as a result of treatment intervention. For example, a patient with back pain must demonstrate altered movement patterns that result in protection from reinjury, or a patient with a traumatic brain injury demonstrates correction of balance in stance and no longer requires supervision. Assessment of motor learning and sustained performance is essential for validating the treatment approach and justifying further physical therapy services.[52–54]

The initial FOR and subsequent FOR document the value of physical therapy services to your patients as well as payers. The FOR approach guides the therapist in reporting the clinical reasoning processes, which address the functional consequence of the underlying problems. The functional outcome report allows you to project clinical reasoning that is clear, logical, and understandable to the reader. Regardless of the complexity of the patient's condition, the therapist can organize clinical observations through this process. It provides a mechanism to clearly communicate treatment strategies which justify treatment intervention and lead to predictable functional outcomes.

In summary the six steps of the FOR process are

1. Establishing patient needs: reason for referral
2. Analyzing performance: identifying and reporting functional limitations
3. Identifying clinical impression: physical therapy assessment
4. Postulating relationships between impairment and performance, leading to identifying therapy problems
5. Predicting a functional outcome: functional outcome goals
6. Devising a treatment strategy: Treatment plan with rationale

Now test your knowledge of the concepts. A completed case study with documentation using the FOR method, and a partially completed sample case study you can use to practice your assessment and documentation skills, follow the test.

REFERENCES

1. Swanson GH: *The functional outcome report* (Design Document). Long Beach, Calif, 1990, Swanson and Company.
2. Weed LL: *Medical records, medical education, and patient care: the problem oriented record as a basic tool.* Chicago, 1971, Year Book.
3. Weed LL, Zimny NJ: The problem-oriented system, problem-knowledge coupling, and clinical decision making, *Phys Ther* 7:565–568, 1989.
4. Swanson GH: Introduction to outcomes management, *Phys Ther Today*, Spring 1991, pp 68–72.
5. Swanson GH: Use of cost data, provider experience, and clinical guidelines in the transition to managed care, *J Insurance Med* 23:70–74, 1991.
6. Swanson GH, Manella K, Foto M: ICIDH codes: a way to report physical therapy outcomes, World Congress of Physical Therapy, London, 1991.
7. Jette AM: Diagnosis and classification by physical therapists: a special communication, *Phys Ther* 69:967–969, 1989.
8. *Competencies in Physical Therapy: An Analysis of Practice*, Washington, D.C., 1977, APTA and Courseware, Inc.
9. *HCFA Intermediary Manual, Medical Review Guidelines*, Transmittal 79: Out-Patient Physical Therapy and CORF's, Baltimore, August 1988, HCFA.
10. Watts NT: Clinical decision analysis, *Physical Therapy* 69:569–576, 1989.
11. Callahan D: Allocating health resources. *Hastings Cent Rep* April/May 1988, pp 14–20.
12. Eddy D: Practice Policies: Where Do They Come From? *JAMA* 263:1265–1275, 1990. (Series: Clinical decision making: from theory to practice.)
13. Purtilo RB: Saying "no" to patients for cost-related reasons: alternatives for the physical therapist, *Phys Ther* 68:1243–1247, 1988.
14. Prevention of injury-related disability. In Pope AM Tarlov AR, editors: *Disability in America: toward a national agenda for prevention*, Washington, D.C., 1991, National Academy Press, pp 147–183.
15. Kramon G: Taking a scalpel to health costs, *New York Times*, January 8, 1989.
16. Gray HG, Field MJ, editors: *Controlling costs and changing patient care?, the role of utilization management*, Washington, D.C., 1989, National Academy Press.
17. Leaf A: Cost effectiveness as a criterion for medicare coverage. *N Engl J Med* 321:898–900, 1989.
18. Blue Cross of California: The cost of therapy services to the Medicare program May 1990.
19. Blue Cross of California: Classification of out-patient therapy services: economic aspects, June 1990.
20. Blue Cross of California: The definition of functional outcome (Prospective Payment of Therapy Services series), April 1991.
21. Wilson DJ, Baker LL, Craddock JA: Functional test for the hemiparetic upper extremity, *Am J Occup Ther* 38:159–164, 1984.
22. Yakura JS, Waters RL, Adkins RH: Predicting gait performance in SCI. Presented at American Physical Therapy Association, Boston, June 1991.

23. Linton SJ, Kamwendo K: Low back schools: a critical review, *Phys Ther* 67:1375–1383, 1987.
24. Fordyce WE et al: Acute Back Pain: A Control-Group Comparison of Behavioral vs. Traditional Management Methods, *J Behav Med* 9:127–140, 1986.
25. Bouter LM: How to assess the effect of physiotherapy: on the importance of developing clinimetric indices, World Congress of Physical Therapy, London, 1991.
26. Deyo RA et al: A controlled trial of transcutaneous electrical nerve stimulation (TENS) and exercise for chronic low back pain, *N Engl J Med* 322:1627–1634, 1990.
27. Allen C, Earhart CA: *Treatment goals for cognitive and physical disability.* Rockville, Md., American Occupational Therapy Association, 1992.
28. Kaufert JM: Functional ability indices: measurement problems in assessing their validity, *Arch Phys Med Rehabil* 64:260–266, 1983.
29. Jette AM, Cleary PD: Functional disability assessment, *Phys Ther* 67:1854–1859, 1987.
30. Schoening HA, Iversen IA: Numerical scoring of self-care status: a study of the Kenny self-care evaluation, *Arch Phys Med Rehabil* 49:221–229, 1968.
31. Mahoney FI, Barthel DW: Functional evaluation: the Barthel index. *Maryland State Med J* 61–63, 1965.
32. Liang H, Jette AM, Measuring functional ability in chronic arthritis, *Arthritis Rheum* 24:80–86, 1981.
33. Jette AM, Deniston OL: Inter-observer reliability of a functional status assessment instrument, *J Chronic Dis* 31:573–580, 1978.
34. Jette AM: Functional capacity evaluation: an empirical approach, *Arch Phys Med Rehabil* 61:85–89, 1980.
35. Reynolds WJ, Rushing WA, Miles DL: The validation of a function status index, *J Health Soc Behav* 15:271–288, 1974.
36. Feinstein AR, Josephy BR, Wells CK: Scientific and clinical problems in indexes of functional disability, *Ann Intern Med* 105:413–420, 1986.
37. *Western physical performance analysis* (Guidebook). Tustin, Calif, Western Neuro Care Center.
38. Granger C et al: Advances in functional assessment for medical rehabilitation. *Top Geriatric Rehabil* 1:59–74, 1986.
39. Tarlov AR et al: The Medical outcomes study: an application of methods for monitoring the results of medical care. *JAMA* 262:925–930, 1989.
40. Bohannon RW: Objective measures, *Phys Ther* 69:590–593, 1989.
41. Ellwood P: Shattuck Lecture, Outcomes management: a technology of patient experience. *N Engl J Med* 318:1549–1556, 1988.
42. *International classification of impairments, disabilities, and handicaps.* Geneva, 1980, World Health Organization.
43. Guccione AA: Physical therapy diagnosis and the relationship between impairments and function, *Phys* 71:499–504, 1991.
44. Jette AM: Diagnosis and classification by physical therapists: a special communication, *Phys Ther* 69:967–969, 1989.

45. Nagi SZ: *Disability and rehabilitation.* Columbus, 1969, Ohio State University Press.
46. Sahrmann SA: Diagnosis by the physical therapist—a prerequisite for treatment, *Phys Ther,* 68:1703–1706, 1988.
47. Schenkman M, Butler RB: A model for multisystem evaluation, interpretation, and treatment of individuals with neurologic dysfunction, *Phys Ther* 69:538–547, 1989.
48. Harris BA, Dyrek DA: A model of orthopaedic dysfunction for clinical decision making in physical therapy practice, *Phys Ther* 69:548–553, 1989.
49. Ottenbacher KJ: *Evaluating clinical change: strategies for occupational and physical therapists,* Baltimore, 1986, Williams & Wilkins.
50. Winstein CJ, Knecht HG, editors: Movement science (special series), *Phys Ther,* volumes 70–71, 1990–1991.
51. Winstein CJ: Knowledge of results and motor learning, implications for physical therapy, *Phys Ther* 71:140–149, 1991.
52. Naliboff BD et al: Comprehensive assessment of chronic low back pain patients and controls: physical abilities, level of activity, psychological adjustment and pain perception, *Pain* 23:121–134, 1985.
53. Manos PA, Schenkman M: Physical therapy management of a geriatric individual with neurological and pulmonary dysfunction: a case analysis, *Top Geriatric Rehabil* (in press).
54. Talmage EW, Collins GA: Physical abilities after head injury: a retrospective study, *Phys Ther* 63:2010–2017, 1983.

TEST YOUR KNOWLEDGE

1. What is functional outcome?

2. What does a payer expect me to report?

3. The Functional Outcome Report (FOR) model includes six major steps. Name each step and describe its major purpose.

4. What relationship does the clinical reasoning process described in Chapter 3 have to the FOR model?

5. Your patient has shown some improvement over the past 3 weeks in pain control, muscle strength, and joint mobility. You are concerned as to whether the patient has shown sufficient improvement. How would you evaluate this?

6. Regardless of the model of functional outcome reporting you use, it should include several concepts. Name them.

7. What is the major reason for the physical therapist to thoroughly investigate patient complaints prior to examining the patient or developing a treatment strategy?

8. Is it possible for a patient to complete a course of treatment and still experience residual impairment and disability, yet have a meaningful functional outcome?

9. Functional assessment tests are controversial in the literature. Questions have been raised regarding their validity, reliability, and meaningfulness. Name some of the problems you may encounter when using these tests.

10. Describe the three parameters you should use when rating tasks.

11. When establishing functional outcomes, what things should you consider to assure that your predictions are credible?

12. What must performance testing demonstrate?

TEST YOUR KNOWLEDGE ANSWER SHEET

1. Functional outcome is a comprehensive and predictable set of specific functional activities and/or tasks that you and the patient agree are most important for the patient to accomplish within a given time.
2. The payer wants to know about functional outcome, not range of motion charts, manual muscle tests, or neurologic scores.
3. The six major steps in a FOR model are
   a. Establishing patient needs: reporting reason for referral
   b. Analyzing performance: identifying and reporting functional limitations
   c. Identifying clinician impression: physical therapy assessment
   d. Postulating relationships between impairment and performance: identifying problems
   e. Predicting a functional outcome: functional outcome goals
   f. Devising a treatment strategy: treatment plan with rationale
4. This model assists the therapist to apply clinical reasoning to determine both the underlying cause and functional consequences of the disorder. It allows you to distinguish the concepts of diagnosis and impairment from functional consequence of the disorder.
5. You need to compare the patient's performance of the target activity or functional task selected during your initial evaluation with the patient's current status, then assess whether the change in status is meaningful, utilitarian, and sustainable.
6. The concepts that should be incorporated into all FOR models are:
   a. It should rely on observable, testable patient function over time.
   b. It should relate to any therapy model or setting.
   c. It should allow the physical therapist to apply *clinical reasoning* to determine both the underlying cause and the functional consequence of the disorder.
   d. It should distinguish the concepts of diagnosis and impairment from the functional consequence of the disorder.
   e. It should permit more accurate useful prediction of outcomes, necessary in a cost-containment and managed care health care system.
   f. It should provide patients and therapists with more realistic, meaningful objectives.
   g. It should provide a rationale for requesting payment of services during the necessary course of physical therapy care.
7. Unless a complete analysis is made of the patient's complaints in terms of need and priority of function, the therapist will find it difficult to determine when the goals have been achieved. One way to assure that this analysis occurs is to use a systematic and routine set of interview questions.

8. Yes. It is not unusual for patients to leave therapy with residual impairment or disability and still function in a meaningful way. For example, a patient with reduced range of motion or muscle strength can have a functional outcome of independent ambulation with a walker in the home environment.

9. Some of the questions regarding validity, reliability, and meaningfulness are centered around whether the tests assess capacity or performance, capability, or disability. Does a test control for devices or motivation? What is the effect of the rater on the score? How meaningful is a generic inventory of activities to all patients? Are you actually assessing level of care or level of performance, and can the functional test be used repeatedly to obtain valid results?

10. The three parameters to use when rating tasks are:
    a. *tolerance:* Can the task be completed once?
    b. *endurance:* can the task be repeated, and how often within a given time?
    c. *performance response:* Are speed and accuracy at the desired level?

11. You should consider function, that is, state the activities or tasks that are most meaningful to the patient and/or caregiver. Consider predicting the outcome by describing the level of physical assistance, severity of limitation, and/or task modification for each function that the patient will achieve at the end of the course of therapy. Develop short-term goals, that is, goals considered to represent what the patient will achieve at the end of the current billing period, referral period, or other meaningful interval. Set long-term goals that describe what will ultimately be achieved by the time the patient is discharged.

12. The major purpose of subsequent reporting is to demonstrate the validity and effectiveness of the predicted outcome. It is to report sustained change during the course of therapy. It requires documenting test-retest findings. This testing must demonstrate that the patient has learned new movement behavior and therefore has advanced or improved in function as a result of treatment intervention.

PRACTICE CASE STUDY: ORTHOPEDIC DYSFUNCTION

A patient has a history of degenerative joint disease of the spine. The patient recently took a trip by airplane, which required prolonged sitting for most of a 7-hour flight. Afterward she complained of pain during walking and was experiencing difficulty in caring for herself. She was referred to you for evaluation and treatment intervention. During the evaluation you observe that the patient demonstrates considerable restriction of function in performing a variety of ambulation and mobility activities. She specifically demonstrates restricted movement of the thoracic and lumber spine and is unable to attain a neutral position, doing so only with external support. She exhibits kyphotic posture when performing postural activities. Joint analysis indicates hard end-feel secondary to long-term osteoarthritis; pain with rotation, indicating local inflammatory response; and shortened length of surrounding soft tissue at T-6 to T-10. Muscle testing reveals weakness of the lower extremity and trunk musculature of good minus. She is unable to maintain erect posture or improved posture greater than 30 seconds without verbal cuing or repositioning.

To justify your treatment strategy for reporting purposes, you need to examine the following factors of orthopedic dysfunction in relation to the patient's function: tissue nutrition, mechanical-tissue load, soft-tissue restriction or lengthening, and motor control. A complete detailed assessment of causal and residual impairments will provide a basis for determining how those impairments will impact on the patient's functional outcome. The following is an example of how the impairment model should be used to apply clinical reasoning in a FOR model for this case study.

FOR REPORT FOR ORTHOPEDIC DYSFUNCTION MODEL

Patient complaint	Reason for referral	
Patient has history of degenerative joint disease of the spine. Since recent airplane flight requiring prolonged sitting (most of 7 hours), patient reports pain during walking, difficulty in caring for self.	Patient's ability to care for self in community, specifically shopping and household management, are limited secondary to mobility tolerance.	
Performance analysis	**Functional Limitation**	
Patient demonstrates restricted postural and gait disorders during various ambulation and mobility activities.	*Activity*	*Current Status*
	Sitting	Unable without intense pain.
	Sidelying	Unable without moderate pain.
	Even terrain ambulation	Able for 10 ft without pain, 25 ft with tolerable pain.
	Uneven terrain ambulation	Unable; occasionally can manage single step.
	Stair climbing	Limited to five without residual pain.

FOR Rᴇᴘᴏʀᴛ ꜰᴏʀ Oʀᴛʜᴏᴘᴇᴅɪᴄ Dʏꜱꜰᴜɴᴄᴛɪᴏɴ Mᴏᴅᴇʟ **(cont.).**

Clinical impression based on tests of impairment and dysfunction	PT assessment
Patient has restricted movement of thoracic and lumbar spine. Able to attain neutral position, but only with external support, causing kyphotic posture during postural activities. Joint analysis indicates hard end-feel secondary to long-term inflammatory response, shortened length of surrounding soft tissue of T-6 to T-10. Patient demonstrates weakness of lower extremity and trunk muscle grade of "good minus" (G⁻); is unable to maintain erect posture or improved posture for more than 30 sec without verbal cuing or repositioning.	Medical diagnosis of acute episode of DJD further defined to include capsular involvement from T-7 to L-5.

Relationship of impairment to activity restriction	Therapy problems
Forward flexion of the thoracic spine causes impingement of local soft tissue; continued flexion in sitting and sidelying maintains impingement. Weight bearing, as in walking, requires control of thoracic spine in extension, which patient is unable to maintain.	1. Thoracic segmental mobility limited; hypomobile in extension 2. Thoracic movement; patient virtually unable to coordinate extension on own; flexion occurs 2 to 3 degrees, secondary to pain and stiffness.

Predicted functional outcome goals

Expect residual loss in thoracic/lumbar joint motion. Reducing capsular inflammation will ease motion, allowing slow but independent upright mobility within 2 to 3 weeks.

Functional outcome goals

Activity	Target Performance Status	Due Date
1. Pain-free sitting	15 min	14 days
2. Pain-free sidelying	Up to 2 hr	7 days
3. Even terrain ambulation	1 hr pain free	7 days
4. Uneven terrain ambulation	Pain tolerable 10–15 ft	14 days
5. Stair climbing	15 stairs pain free	21 days

Treatment strategy	Treatment plan
Monitor involved spinal joints following reduction in capsular inflammation. Increase lower extremity and trunk strength to reduce stress on spine during upright tasks.	1. Anti-inflammatory modalities for both local control of swelling and neurophysiologic effect to control pain. 2. Instruct in lower extremity and trunk exercises; supervise exercises until inflammation is eliminated. 3. Integrate improved trunk posture into movement during upright activities to minimize further joint involvement and improve overall mobility.

Now that you have reviewed the sample case study using the FOR method, practice your clinical decision skills, remembering the principles of the orthopedic dysfunction model presented in Chapter 3. Practice report writing by filling in the missing information in the following case study. It may be helpful on completion of this exercise to carefully review the neurological impairment model "Example of Functional Disability Following Stroke," which appears in Appendix II–B.

PRACTICE CASE STUDY: NEUROLOGIC DYSFUNCTION

A patient is referred to you with a medical diagnosis of acute cerebrovascular accident (CVA) with parietal lobe involvement (right-sided CVA). The patient has been recently discharged to the home environment and is being seen as an outpatient. The caregiver reports that the patient is unable to ambulate safely around the room because of poor balance and therefore is not attempting activities of daily living independently. The patient has difficultly with balance while sitting, attempting to stand, and walking. On evaluation you validate the patient's balance problems in that sitting and standing balance requires stand-by supervision, and ambulation in the parallel bars requires moderate assistance on the straightaway and maximum assistance on turns. The patient also fatigues quickly when attempting ambulation activities. Tests you perform indicate hypotonia of the trunk and lower left extremity, with reduced motor control of the left lower extremity, trunk, and left upper quadrant. There is left lower extremity neglect during upright activity. Complete the clinical reasoning process and FOR report for an initial evaluation on this patient. A form is provided at the end of this chapter.

NEUROLOGIC CASE STUDY	FOR REPORT ITEM	
Patient complaint Caregiver reports patient unable to to safely ambulate about room following right-sided CVA.	**Reason for referral** Patient was an independent ambulator about home and community. Now requires physical assistance from spouse to ambulate about home; community ambulation not attempted.	
Performance analysis Patient demonstrates faulty balance in sit-to-stand, sit-to-sit, standing, and assisted gait activities; unassisted activities not attempted because of safety considerations.	**Functional limitation** *(Identify the status of activities based on the limitations listed.*	
	Activity	*Current Status*
	Sitting	
	Sit-to-stand	
	Sit-to-sit	
	Standing	
	Ambulate in parallel bars	

Neurologic Case Study (cont.)

Clinical impression based on tests of impairment and dysfunction	PT assessment
Patient has hypotonia of the trunk and left lower extremity neglect during upright activity, and limited endurance. Motor tests reveal:	Medical diagnosis of acute CVA with parietal lobe involvement is further defined to include the following:
Relationship of impairment to activity restriction	**Therapy problems**
There is a direct relationship between the patient's _____ _____ and _____ mobility. Activities related to problems include: _____ , _____ , _____ . Lack of ability in these areas result in what kind of of restrictions for caregiver and patient? _____	1. Loss of upright trunk control 2. Inadequate weightbearing on left lower limb 3. Minimal motor learning potential

(Predict the amount of time required to reach the specific level of activities based on information provided below.)

Predicted functional outcome	Functional outcome goals		
Activity	*Target Performance Status*		*Due date*
			15 days
Unsupported sitting			
Supported sitting	Independent		_____
Sit-to-stand			15 days
Sit-to-sit			
Stand	Assisted		Current
Ambulate in parallel bars	Supervised		_____ days
			21 days

Treatment strategy	Treatment plan with rationale
Increase duration of unassisted unsupported sitting (5 min) and standing (30 sec). Instruct caregiver in ambulation and transfer techniques. Provide three sessions of _____ _____ activities to ascertain motor learning capabilities.	1. 2. Caregiver instructed safe ambulation and transfers for home 3. Trial during upright activities to monitor effect on faulty balance

CLINICAL REASONING PROCESS	FOR REPORT ITEM		
Establish patient need	**Reason for referral**		
Analyze patient performance (assess activity restrictions)	**Functional limitation**		
	Activity	*Current Status*	
Identify clinical impressions (complete tests of impairment and dysfunction)	**PT assessment**		
Postulate relationship between impairment and performance	**Therapy problems**		
Predict functional outcome	**Functional outcome goals**		
	Activity	*Target Performance*	*Due date*
Devise treatment strategy	**Treatment plan with rationale**		

CHAPTER 5

Applying Functional Outcome Assessment to Medicare Documentation

Linda Esposto, PT

Key Concepts

- Purpose of Medicare
- Definition of skilled physical therapy in Medicare Parts A and B
- The Medicare evaluation
- Medicare monthly summary
- Medicare discharge summary
- Medicare appeal process

PURPOSE OF MEDICARE

The federal government has been a major payer of health care since the early 1960s. Over the past 2 decades the design of the health care delivery system has moved the nation closer to managed care concepts. Many of these concepts emerged as a result of congressional amendments to the Social Security Act during the 1960s. Further amendments mandated prospective payment practices as a mechanism for containing health care cost, especially for beneficiaries who were eligible for *Medicare* supplemental coverage. The number of citizens eligible for Medicare has increased with the general aging of the nation's population. Prospective payment has been in place since 1986 and has become the prevailing model for reimbursement. There has been a continual shift from fee for service reimbursement to prospective payment based on care that is determined reasonable and medically necessary. The focus on outcome has moved from treatment of disability and impairment to one of functionally related outcome. All providers must be familiar with the current regulations that guide reimbursement activities under this federally subsidized program. To document and develop treatment interventions resulting in successful reimbursement, one must understand the history and purpose of the Medicare programs and be knowledgeable about required documentation. This Chapter focuses on these aspects of Medicare entitlement and the regulations related to physical therapy services.

The Medicare program was established in 1966 as a federal health insurance program. Persons over age 65 and disabled persons of any age who meet specific medical criteria are eligible for admission to the program. The program is administered by the Health Care Financing Administration (HCFA) of the United States Department of Health and Human Services. This government agency contracts with private insurance organizations to administer the Medicare program. There are two types of Medicare insurance entities with whom the government contracts: **intermediaries** and **carriers.** Intermediaries are responsible for claims submitted on the behalf of a client by a hospital and other providers of services. Carriers are responsible for claims submitted on behalf of the client by a physician and other health care providers. Intermediaries are cost-based providers; carriers are charge-based providers. Regardless of who initiates the claim, the carrier or intermediary responsible for processing the individual claims makes determinations based on the Medicare law as to whether the claim is **reasonable and necessary** for payment in the Medicare system.[1] Since the interpretation of the Medicare law is done by either a carrier or an intermediary, one may find differences in payment depending on which entity is processing the claim. As providers of service, physical therapists should be familiar with the carrier or intermediary that is processing claims and have general knowledge of the process of interpretation.

Medicare has two components: Medicare Part A and Medicare Part B. **Medicare Part A** is hospital insurance; **Medicare Part B** is medical insurance. The hospital insurance (Part A) covers inpatient hospital care, inpatient skilled nursing facilities, home health care, and hospice care. A person or spouse who is 65 years or older, has been employed, and is eligible to receive social security benefits is eligible for Part A benefits. The medical insurance (Part B) covers physician services, outpatient hospital services, durable medical equipment, and other medical services and supplies that hospital insurance does not cover. To receive Medicare Part B, a person must meet the previous criteria and pay a monthly premium. Both Part A and

Part B include annual deductibles for which the patient is responsible prior to payment from Medicare program funds. The provider can determine the type of insurance coverage the patient has by looking at the patient's Medicare card. The card will have the words "hospital," "medical," or both printed on it, and also the effective date on which the person was eligible to receive benefits. Each component of Medicare will be discussed in detail later in this chapter. Table 5–1 illustrates the two major components of Medicare coverage, eligibility requirements, services covered by each component, and the insurance entity responsible for review of claims.

DEFINITION OF SKILLED PHYSICAL THERAPY

Accurate and complete documentation is an integral part of a physical therapist's overall performance responsibilities in patient care. It creates a record of the patient's progress and presents the rationale for reimbursement. The physical therapist must be an expert in documentation as well as in other aspects of patient evaluation and treatment planning.

When dealing with Medicare patients, it is imperative that the therapist who evaluates these patients read and clearly understand the Medicare regulations pertinent to physical therapy intervention. Every physical therapy facility involved in treating Medicare patients should maintain a copy of these regulations, found in the *Health Insurance Manual (HIM)* published by HCFA. There are two sections in this manual that are important to physical therapists and with which they should become familiar. These are listed

TABLE 5–1.

SUMMARY OF MEDICARE COVERAGE*

Criteria for Eligibility	Insurance Coverage	Claims Reviewer†
Part A: *Hospital* Must be eligible for Social Security Must pay annual deductible prior to Medicare payment	Inpatient hospital care Inpatient skilled nursing care Home health care Hospice care	Intermediary

Part B: *Medical*
Must pay monthly premium
Must pay deductible prior to Medicare
   payment
	Physician services
	Other medical services
	Supplies and services not covered
	   by Part A
	Outpatient hospital services
	Durable medical equipment
		Intermediary and/or carrier

*Patient's Medicare card identifies type of coverage, that is, hospital or medical or both.
†If cost based, will be an intermediary.

under the headings of "Therapy" and are entitled "Coverage of Services" and "Billing Procedures."

Many providers and persons eligible for Medicare insurance assume that the purpose of Medicare is to pay for all medical needs of the individual. Providers and Medicare recipients often do not understand that the concept of Medicare was not intended to provide basic overall insurance, but rather supplemental insurance. They are unaware that there are written regulations which identify the criteria that must be met before a specific service claim will be paid. Recipients often fail to understand that if they want broader and more comprehensive health care coverage beyond what is allowed under the Medicare program, it must be purchased from a private insurance source.

It is also important that the provider of care understand that those agents responsible for the operational or procedural aspects of the Medicare program—intermediaries or carriers—do not dictate to the provider whom to treat, but rather determine which patients meet the criteria for payment. In order to present documentation in a manner that will justify payment of the claim, providers must have an understanding of the Medicare criteria used to make such determination for eligibility for payment.

The Components of Medicare

Medicare Part A

The Medicare program has specific criteria for Part A eligibility for each type of medical facility. The admitting personnel or the utilization review committee of the facility reviews the individual's medical history and determines if the level of care qualifies the individual for admittance to the facility as an inpatient. The physical therapist may or may not play a role in this decision. Regardless of whether one has a role in the determination process, one should read the Medicare regulations, especially the section entitled "Coverage of Services," which pertains to the type of facility in which one practices. Generally the determining criteria for admittance to a facility under Medicare Part A as it relates to physical therapy is that *the patient's condition warrants such intense therapy that it is **reasonable and necessary** to furnish care on an inpatient daily basis rather than an outpatient basis.*[1]

Once the patient is admitted for Medicare Part A coverage, the medical documentation, including the physical therapy evaluation and progress notes, will be the justification for the inpatient level of care. It is important to note that Part A therapy can only be received in a hospital, skilled facility, and home health setting.

Medicare Part B

Medicare Part B provides reimbursement for outpatient physical therapy. Outpatient therapy is defined as *service given to a patient who is under the care of a physician and has a plan of care written by a physician or therapist who is treating the patient.*[1] The plan includes the type, amount, and duration of the physical therapy treatment. The Part B phase of therapy is usually not as intense as that under Part A and therefore does not require treatment on a daily basis or on an inpatient basis. Therapy under Medicare Part B can be received in an outpatient hospital, skilled facility, home health agency, or rehabilitation agency or in the setting of an independent practice.

Documentation for physical therapy under Medicare Part A or Part B is the same.

Criteria for Eligibility for Physical Therapy Services.—According to the Medicare guidelines,[1] for a patient to be eligible for coverage, two criteria must be met. The services must

1. Relate directly and specifically to an active written treatment program established by a physician or a physical therapist providing the services.
2. Be reasonable and necessary to the treatment of an individual illness or injury.

The first criterion must be met through an active written program. This program is the evaluation which details the plan of care. The second criterion is met by including in the evaluation the four conditions cited in the Medicare guidelines which define the terms "reasonable and necessary." These are described in the following

Conditions of "Reasonable and Necessary" Care.—The four conditions that define reasonable and necessary care are the crux for determining the *eligible status* of the treatment. As stated in the Medicare guidelines,[1] the four conditions are as follows:

1. The services must be considered under the accepted standards of the medical practice to be specific and effective treatment for the patient's condition.

2. The services must be of such level of complexity and sophistication or the condition of the patient such that the services required can be safely

and effectively performed only by a qualified physical therapist or under his/her supervision.

3. There must be an expectation that the condition will improve significantly in a reasonable (and generally predictable) period of time, based on the assessment made by the physician, of the patient's *restoration potential* after any needed consultation with the qualified physical therapist, or the services must be necessary to the establishment of a safe and effective maintenance program required in connection with a specific disease state.

4. The amount, frequency and duration of the services must be reasonable.

Many physical therapists become frustrated over the lack of specificity in interpreting these four conditions and the fact that they are vague and allow for wide interpretation. To avoid adverse judgments based on this vagueness, the therapist must be able to write in a manner that is concise and meets all of the conditions of reasonable and necessary. One way to do this is by reviewing the documentation and answering the following questions as they relate directly to the four conditions that define reasonable and necessary:

1. Is the service documented an accepted treatment based on the patient's condition? For example, biofeedback is a covered modality under Medicare when it is used for "muscle reeducation." It is not covered when it is used for "relief of muscle tension."

2. Does the documentation demonstrate that the judgment, knowledge, and skills of the physical therapist were needed to perform the service rather that being performed by ancillary personnel? *Skill* is the *key word* in answering this question. For example, heat or cold modalities used as the *only* treatment and applied by the *physical therapist* would not be coverable. However, if the heat or cold were given *in conjunction with therapeutic exercise,* it would be coverable. Therapeutic exercise is included in the list of *skilled therapies* in the Medicare regulations.

3. Does the documentation make clear that the physical therapy services provided produce a "functional or measurable gain" and do the services provided occur within a time frame which is "reasonable?" For example, if the documentation were to read, "Pain is less and the patient feels better after treatment of ultrasound and exercise," the service would not be coverable. However, if the documentation were, "Pain has decreased from 9 to 5 (with 10 being constant pain) after 1 week of ultrasound and exercise," the service would be coverable. Remember, a statement must be made which

uses *measurable and objective terminology.* This latter example is objective and also describes progress in measurable terms.

4. Does the documentation indicate that the condition of the patient supports the decision regarding the frequency and duration of the treatment plan? For example, if the documentation read "daily therapy for 4 to 6 weeks" it would not be coverable. If the documentation read "Daily therapy for 4 to 6 weeks due to the acuteness of a CVA" and this statement was followed by *a list of goals directly related to and/or reasonable for the patient's condition,* it would be coverable.

The underlying criterion for achieving approval or eligibility for reimbursement of physical therapy services is *clear documentation that demonstrates a relationship between the patient condition and treatment which is "reasonable and necessary" and requires the skill of a professional physical therapist.* This criterion pervades all types of documentation, including the evaluation, the monthly summary, or the discharge summary. Table 5–2 is a summary of the criteria for reasonable and necessary services and the questions that the documentation must answer.

MEDICARE EVALUATION

The purpose of the evaluation is to establish the baseline information needed to assess the rehabilitation potential of the patient. For the reviewer to make a determination regarding this potential, it is imperative that,

TABLE 5–2.

EFFECT OF THE CRITERIA FOR REASONABLE AND NECESSARY SERVICES ON DOCUMENTATION

Criteria	Questions Documentation Must Answer
1. Services are based on accepted standard that is *specific and effective* for condition	Is service documented accepted treatment based on condition?
2. Service is at level of complexity or patient's condition requires that a physical therapist perform the services in order for it to be safely and effectively rendered	Does the service require the judgment, knowledge, and skill of the physical therapist or could ancillary personnel do it?
3. Expectation that outcome will occur or physical therapist's skill is required to establish a safe and effective maintenance program based on disease state	Is there demonstration that a *functional or measurable* gain have occurred? Is the therapist's skills required to develop a maintenance program?
4. Amount, frequency and duration are reasonable	Is there a strong indication that the patient's condition supports the frequency, intensity and duration of treatment?

through documentation, care is taken to set realistic goals that are measurable for determining patient progress. The three major elements of the evaluation are the justification for the referral, assessment of the findings, and the treatment plan and goals.

Element of the Evaluation

Justification for Referral

There are three critical elements within the concept of justification for referral that need to be addressed: the reason for the referral, the pertinent medical history, and the previous functional level of the patient.

Reason for Referral.—The first element to address in an evaluation is the need or reason for the physical therapy service or for the justification for the referral. Although it is assumed that the reason for a referral is most often reflected in the diagnosis (such as a fractured hip), a more accurate description of the patient's functional limitations (e.g., numerous falls that result in inability to ambulate safely in the home) should be included in the documentation. The statement of reason must be made to assure that it is obvious to the reviewer that the *professional judgment* of the physical therapist is needed. In the example above, the reason for the referral (numerous falls that result in inability to function in the home setting) clearly indicates that the judgment of the physical therapist is needed to "evaluate" why the falls are occurring and to determine or identify the rehabilitation potential of the patient. Always remember that once the reason for the treatment has been established, the therapist should *never lose sight of the reason through the entire course of the evaluation and treatment.* If you lose sight of the purpose, regardless of how well you go through the process, you will not present a successful rationale for reimbursement.

Pertinent Medical History.—The second element of the Medicare evaluation is the gathering of the medical history pertinent to the patient's current medical problem, that is, the problem for which the referral has been made, not the past medical history of the patient. This history should be stated in terms of how the current medical history will affect the treatment of the patient's present condition.

Previous Functional Level.—The third element of the evaluation is the identification and statement of the patient's level of function prior to the current diagnosis and referral. This step is important because the previous level of function provides the foundation on which the therapist can establish realistic goals for the patient. If the prior level is unknown, the therapist should ask the patient for this information. If the patient cannot provide the information, the therapist should assume that a higher level of function existed previously than that currently exhibited by the patient. This assumption is based on the premise that the decreased functional level is the rationale for the referral of the patient for the physical therapy consultation. Also, if the patient received any physical therapy services prior to this evaluation, it should be noted along with the reason why continued therapy is indicated at this time.

In summary, the three elements that should always be included in the part of the evaluation directed at determining the justification for the physical therapy intervention are reasons for referral, pertinent medical history, and level of previous and current function. These elements provide the information the reviewer needs to determine if the treatment or services requested are reasonable and necessary based on the patient's condition.

Assessment of Findings

Once the section of the justification for the referral is completed, the next step in the evaluation process is assessment of the findings. The related documentation establishes the need for the patient to be seen by the physical therapist. One method of reporting these findings is through the use of tests and measurements that are needed to evaluate the patient's rehabilitation potential and that require the skill of the physical therapist. In describing the findings of these tests and measurements, the results should be stated in objective terms and be specific to the diagnosis. It is critical that you show a linkage between the tests/findings/impairments and functional limitation in your documentation. This linkage to function assists the reviewer in understanding the rationale for what you are doing. These findings are the rationale for the need for skilled physical therapy. Examples of appropriate tests and measurements include those measuring range of motion, strength, pain, gait dysfunction, balance, posture, and so forth; these are included in the Medicare regulations. The following are suggested ways to assist the therapist in reporting the clinical findings which result from the tests and measurements in terms that are descriptive and measurable:

1. *Range of motion.*—The use of a ratio of the measured degree of the involved joint over the normal degree of the noninvolved joint is a good way to record a measurable description. *Example:* "Right shoulder displays 70/130 degrees of flexion."

2. *Strength.*—Strength should be graded using numbers and a ratio. The scale of 1 to 5 with 5 as normal and 1 as trace gives the reviewer objec-

tive data. The ratio should be expressed with a number representing the strength of the involved muscle over the number representing the strength of the noninvolved side. *Example:* "The patient's quadriceps strength on the right is 2/5."

3. *Pain.*—Pain should be graded numerically and described in terms of a ratio. It is also important to note pain location, visual assessment of the site of the pain, frequency, distribution, exacerbating factors, and how the pain alters the patient's function. *Example:* "Pain is rated 8/10 with 10 being constant excruciating pain. Inspection of the left knee reveals tenderness to palpation on the medial aspect with a moderate degree of swelling and redness noted. Due to the pain, the patient is no longer able to ambulate independently the distance to the bathroom in her living environment."

4. *Gait.*—The gait should be described. The steppage, speed, posture, and spacing of the base should be mentioned. The therapist should describe the gait by noting how much assistance is needed and what devices are needed. The documentation should also identify how function may be enhanced through improved gait. *Example:* "The patient ambulates with a walker with moderate assist of one person. Patient's gait is slow, upper body is forward flexed. Knees demonstrate increased flexion with exertion. Patient is no longer able to ambulate to and from the dining hall safely."

In your report the patient's clinical findings must document functional loss. The need for physical therapy intervention should be stated, detailing specific conditions such as self-care dependence, mobility dependence, safety dependence, and secondary conditions. A description of these findings must also be in objective terms that will justify the need for the skills of the physical therapist. The following areas at least should be assessed to determine functional levels:

1. *Transfers or bed mobility.*—When assessing transfers or bed mobility, the therapist should describe in the documentation the following: (a) what devices are used; (b) how many people are needed to assist in the transfer; (c) the length of time required for transfer; (d) how intervention will improve transfer or bed mobility so that the patient's involvement in activities of daily living (ADLs) or overall function will increase, for example, "Patient needs moderate assist of one to move supine to sit and perform a transfer from a bed to chair without a device. Patient has never been instructed or attempted transfer with sliding board. The patient's condition indicates the potential to be independent in transfer with a sliding board."

2. *Balance.*—Balance abnormalities should be noted in the objective section of the evaluation. The therapist should distinguish between visual,

perceptual, and muscle problems that affect balance. It should be noted when the patient's balance is affected and how the abnormality alters the patient's function. *Example:* "Patient's sitting balance is fair, and he tends to fall forward in wheelchair. The impaired balance has caused the patient to be unsafe in wheelchair mobility and therefore he is unable to attend outside activities."

3. *Posture.*—Posture may affect the patient's ADLs. A description of posture sitting and standing should be noted. *Example:* "Patient displays severe kyphosis and needs wheelchair adaption to sit safely at bathroom sink to perform morning care."

4. *Chronic Conditions*—Chronic conditions such as degenerative loss of vision in some situations, arthritis, or cardiovascular insufficiency may affect the assessment or goals for the patient. "Patient is legally blind and therefore will always need assistance with ambulation outside her home environment."

5. *Efficiency.*—Measuring endurance so that a patient can improve efficiency should not be overlooked. However, remember, that the *need* for the therapist to accomplish efficiency, not endurance, is important. *Example:* "If the patient can master independent transfer from bed to wheelchair with less energy expenditure, he will be able to be left in his home unattended during the day and still have the energy to perform self-care."

In summary, the assessment section of the Medicare evaluation justifies the need for the patient to be seen by the physical therapist in order to *determine the potential for rehabilitation*. It also demonstrates that the skill of the therapist is necessary to document the findings obtained from tests and measurements used to determine the level of functional loss experienced by the patient.

Treatment Plan and Goals

The next step in the evaluation process is to determine the treatment plan and goals for the patient. These must be based on and related to the findings of the evaluation. The plan should include a list of therapy modalities that will be administered to the patient. These treatments must be appropriate for the condition of the patient. The plan must include the frequency and duration of treatment and relate directly to the physical therapy goals. As discussed previously, it is important to reasonably estimate a termination date. It is always important to the reviewer to know when therapy is expected to end. The goals must be reasonable for the patient's diagnosis and environment. A *measurable* and *functional* goal should be noted so that the reviewer will be able to judge the potential for improvement and whether it will be obtained in a "reasonable and necessary" time frame. *Example:* "To increase quadriceps strength from 2/5 to 3+/5 to enable the patient to use a safe gait with the walker. A safe gait will enable patient to ambulate a functional distance in his living environment so that he is independent in bathroom activities. The plan will be 'daily therapeutic exercises for 2 weeks to the lower left extremity, followed by gait training with a walker.' "

In summary, when documenting always remember all of the elements of the evaluation process are necessary to justify the need for a physical therapist's skill for the consultation. *After writing an evaluation, you should read it as if you were the reviewer.* In your review, ask what skill is needed and whether this skill is documented concisely and objectively. The major elements of the review process are summarized in Table 5–3.

Medicare Evaluation for One-Time Consultation

In many cases, the evaluation may be a one-time consultation. In this situation, the evaluation should follow the method of documentation just reviewed except in documenting the treatment plan and goals. Instead of a plan with goals, the consultation documentation should note that a physical therapist has made recommendations, taught the patient, or initiated changes in the patient's current program. The Medicare regulations list assessment as an accepted physical therapy treatment; therefore, the consul-

TABLE 5–3.

RESPONSE IN DOCUMENTATION TO THREE MAJOR ELEMENTS OF MEDICARE REVIEW PROCESS

Requirement	Documentation
Initial evaluation	
Justification for referral	Diagnosis or statement of *reason for referral*
Pertinent medical history	History pertinent to treating current condition
Previous functional level	Statement about level of functioning prior to current diagnosis and referral
Assessment of findings to establish need for physical therapy	
Tests and measurements (range of motion, strength, pain, gait)	Describe findings that assess condition; state in objective and in functional terms specific to diagnosis
Transfers, bed mobility, balance, posture, chronic conditions, efficacy	Document functional loss
Treatment plan and goals based on findings	
Must be objective, measurable, and functional to demonstrate potential for improvement within a reasonable timeframe	Include lists of modalities, frequency, and relation to goals; must be reasonable for diagnosis and environment; provide an estimated time line for care

tation is reimbursable, if the need for the therapist's skill is clearly documented.[1]

Case Study: Initial Evaluation

Table 5−4 presents a case study that illustrates an initial evaluation, the first element of the review process. This case may or may not qualify for reimbursement under Medicare regulations. As you review the case study, read it as though you were a reviewer who has never seen the patient. This review should allow you to determine if this documentation justifies the need for skilled care according to the condition of the patient and the patient's living environment. Following the case study is a sample format (Table 5−5) that can be used in your clinic to prepare and/or review your documentation.

TABLE 5−4.

Case Study for Assessment of Whether Initial Evaluation Qualifies for Medicare Reimbursement*

Initial Evaluation	Review Steps
Diagnosis: Degenerative joint disease (DJD) in both knees **S:** Patient states, "My knees are bad and I have trouble walking unless someone is with me." She does walk in her room by holding onto furniture.	Reason for referral
O: Patient is an elderly white woman who has a history of DJD. She was previously an independent ambulator with a standard cane and now needs assistance when out of her room. The patient's mental status is alert and oriented × 3, pleasant, and cooperative.	Pertinent medical history
Range of motion: Bilateral upper extremities are WFL; arthritic changes noted in finger joints; bilateral lower extremities are WFL at hips; right knee displays 10 to 100 degrees and left 0 to 100 degrees. *Strength:* Bilateral upper extremities 4/5, right lower 3/5, left lower 3+/5. *Transfer:* Sit-to-stand with difficulty, but independent, using arms to push up from chair; pivot transfers independently. *Ambulation:* Able to ambulate 50 ft with a standard cane with assistance of one; gait is unsteady; attempted ambulation with walker and was able to walk 50 ft with a steady gait unassisted. Needed some verbal cueing for proper walker placement and sequencing.	Prior level of functional return
A: Patient ambulates more safely with a walker for extended distances. Able to use cane in her room along with holding onto furniture. Able to ambulate in hall with walker and nursing supervision.	Assessment of findings
P: Place on maintenance ambulation to supervise safety with walker. Patient may also be supervised by nursing. Should use walker when out of room.	Treatment plan and goals

*SOAP = subjective, objective, assessment, plan.

TABLE 5–5.

SAMPLE FORMAT FOR INITIAL EVALUATION OF MEDICARE PATIENT

Initial evaluation	
Diagnosis:	Review Steps
S:	Justification for referral
O:	Pertinent medical history Prior level of functional return
A:	Assessment of findings
P:	Treatment plan and goals

Critiquing the Evaluation

On completion of the initial evaluation, the therapist should review the evaluation to determine if the key points needed to qualify for reimbursement under Medicare regulations are included in the documentation. The key points are reason for evaluation or referral; medical history and statement of previous level of function; and assessment of findings, with plan and goals.

Reason for Referral

From the case study presented can the reviewer learn the reason for the evaluation? The patient's diagnosis is degenerative joint disease, which is chronic. The evaluation does not mention a recent increase in pain or a description of the joint. Therefore, this diagnosis is not a reimbursable reason for referral. After reading the section noting objective findings, the conclusion should be that the referral was given because of gait dysfunction. Thus "gait dysfunction" is the primary diagnosis, and "DJD" the secondary diagnosis. The reason for the referral is now established.

Medical History/Prior Level of Function

The only medical history listed is the diagnosis of DJD. This is pertinent because the disease could interfere with the patient's ability to ambulate, and noting this supports the reason for evaluation: "gait dysfunction." It is is noted and documented that this patient had previously functioned independently in ambulation with a standard cane in her living environment. Therefore, it is reasonable to assume that she can return to this level of function, as there is no mention of any medical reason that would prevent this type of progression. The medical history and prior level of function are sufficiently documented.

Assessment and Findings

The objective findings should be reviewed. Remember they should present a baseline condition for comparison of further treatment and be specific regarding the reason for the treatment. This case study lacks a description of the need for the expertise of a skilled physical therapist. In essence, the tests and measurements, which are considered skilled therapy, are not sufficient or related to the reason for referral. Remember, the primary reason for referral of this patient is the gait dysfunction, not lack of range or strength. The therapist should document findings that assist in evaluation of the patient's gait. The skills required of the therapist are evaluation and teaching of an appropriate gait for the patient's condition. The key words are *evaluation* and *teach*. The objective findings should describe the gait, noting steppage, posture, balance, assistance, and safety. There should be more discussion of teaching methods, such as verbal and visual cuing, included in the documentation.

Plan/Goals

The goal described is that the patient was taught safe gait with the proper device that would allow her to ambulate functional distances in her environment. Teaching a safe gait with an appropriate device as described in this evaluation is a reasonable goal for the patient. However, the reviewer would have to reach this conclusion on his or her own, as this activity is not stated as a goal. The care plan should be revised to include *a statement not only to place the patient on a maintenance program,* but also to describe *why it was necessary to perform the evaluation.* Such a statement could state, "This evaluation was necessary to determine the safest assistive device for this patient. Patient was instructed in the use of the walker, which was more safe than her current device, a cane. She was instructed to discontinue using the cane. Will monitor patient for 1 week." These changes in documentation make it clear to the reviewer that skilled physical therapy was not only needed, but was actually performed in the intervention of this case. The changes also present a rationale for payment based on the fact that the evaluation was necessary in order to determine the appropriate assistive device and to teach the appropriate use of the device.

MEDICARE MONTHLY SUMMARY

Once the decision is made to treat the patient and to submit the claim to Medicare for reimbursement, the patient's chart must include follow-up documentation. If Medicare requests information on a claim, a monthly summary of progress must be available to accompany the Medicare claim. All follow-up documentation must continue to be developed in objective terms. The summary of the patient's treatment must address three issues: (1) it must justify why physical therapy is indicated; (2) it must show justification for treatment throughout the entire claim period; and (3) it must show why treatment should be continued. The question of why therapy is indicated is addressed by stating the diagnosis or restating the reason for referral and/or continuing treatment. The answer to the question of (why therapy was given) is, "This patient is being seen because of a left hip fracture." The question of why treatment was given throughout the claim period is addressed by the statement of progress in objective and measurable terms. The answer to the question of why treatment was done for the entire treatment period is, "The range and strength of the left hip has improved as follows: range in flexion from 45/120 to 90/120; abduction 10/25 to 20/25; strength in flexion from 2/5 to 3/5; and abduction 2/5 to 3/5. Follow these impairment-based results with a linkage of functional measures. Gait training has progressed from parallel bars with non-weight bearing on the patient's left side and with moderate assistance of two persons, to walker with non-weight bearing with moderate assistance of one." The issue of continuation is addressed by a statement of the unmet goals. The answer to why therapy was continued is, "Therapy will continue daily for 2 weeks to increase the patient's range from flexion 90/120 to 120/120, the strength in flexion from 3/5 to 4/5, and the abduction from 2/5 to 3/5. It is important to continue to link this impairment to functional limitation and outcome. Will progress patient to independent ambulation with walker and progress to other device as physician indicates change in weight-bearing status."

It is important to keep in mind that the monthly summary must demonstrate clearly that significant progress will be obtained in a reasonable time frame and that treatment is necessary for a patient's return to a previous level of function or the maximum functional level attainable for the current condition. A Medicare reviewer may agree that a specific therapy program is reasonable for the condition of the patient, but deny it, based on lack of evidence that the frequency or duration is necessary based on the patient's current environment. In such case, Medicare would reimburse only a portion of the therapy sessions. In conclusion, the content of the monthly summary should show evidence that the therapy administered required "skilled personnel" and that the "goals were realistic for this patient's environment and condition." Table 5–7, which follows the case study, can be used in your clinic to prepare and/or review your documentation.

Case Study: Monthly Summary

The following is a case study of a Medicare monthly summary. Read the summary as though you were a reviewer, to determine if it justifies therapy services, why the patient was treated for the claim period, and why therapy was continued.

TABLE 5–6.

CASE STUDY FOR DOCUMENTATION ANALYSIS

Monthly Summary	Anticipated Reviewer's Questions
Diagnosis: Post-op carpal tunnel and pain	

Monthly Summary	Anticipated Reviewer's Questions
This female resident was evaluated 1 week from this date with diagnosis of post-op carpal tunnel right hand with decreased strength and function on the right. On her arrival in therapy, the right hand and wrist are placed in a whirlpool tank for 20 minutes. She states the whirlpool does not aggravate the condition of the hand, but it is not making it feel any better either. She is also receiving ultrasound to right wrist at 1.5 WPC2 for 5 minutes to alleviate pain and soften scar tissue that resulted from surgery.	Why therapy
Pain: The resident continues to have pain in the wrist that extends through the thumb and the middle finger of the right hand. She states the pain is constant and the medication is not working. Resident rates her pain at 8/10, with 10 being extreme pain.	Why treated throughout period of claim
Range of motion: ROM tests reveal 0–60/90 degrees wrist flexion actively, 60/90 degrees passively; ulnar deviation, 0–20/25 degrees actively, 25/25 degrees passively; radial deviation 15/25 degrees actively, 17/25 degrees passively.	
Strength: In reference to movement and strength, the right wrist is difficult for her to move and thus she is not moving it as well as she should be. She is unable to oppose the thumb to fifth finger, although she is able to oppose to all other fingers. The strength in wrist is 2/5. She is unable to use the hand for any activities of daily living.	
Function: On evaluation, she was ambulating with walker and contact guard of one for functional distances. She was having wrist pain during ambulation, stating that the weight of the walker caused the pain. She was given a very light walker, which did decrease the pain but did not eliminate it. Gait training with a quad cane will eliminate the use of the right hand for ambulation. Resident is unsteady with the cane and tends to lose her balance. Will continue teaching her with quad cane for improved balance and safety. Since the physical therapy was initiated only 1 week ago, the improvements to wrist range and pain levels are minimal.	
Plan: Will be recommended to continue physical therapy at three sessions per week for 4 weeks for whirlpool, ultrasound, and therapeutic exercise to right wrist, followed by gait training with quad cane.	Why therapy continued
Goals: 1. Decrease pain in right wrist from 8/10 to 2/10. 2. Achieve functional R.O.M. to right wrist and achieve increased right wrist strength from 2/5 to 3+/5. With increase in range and strength there will be an increased role in her activities of daily living. 3. Resident will ambulate with quad cane independently for functional distances in her home.	

TABLE 5–7.

SAMPLE FORMAT FOR MONTHLY SUMMARY REPORTS*

Diagnosis: Statement of diagnosis or reason for referral	Why therapy?
Objective data: Statement of progress in objective and functional measurable terms	Why treated throughout period of claim?
Statement of *unmet goals*	Why therapy continued?

*Summary must demonstrate clearly that significant progress will be obtained in a reasonable time and that treatment is necessary for the patient to return to a previous level of function or maximum functional level attainable for the condition.

Critiquing Monthly Summary

This monthly summary includes the necessary objective data to support the reimbursable claim based on the Medicare definitions of *"reasonable and necessary"* (see Table 5–2). The treatment with whirlpool, ultrasound, and therapeutic exercise for this diagnosis is acceptable for the patient's condition under standards of medical practice as defined in the Medicare regulations. The teaching of the quad cane and the therapeutic exercise to the wrist supports the need for skilled therapy because of the level of complexity and sophistication of the therapy procedures. The expectation that the patient will improve significantly is a reasonable goal because the surgery has been recent, no complications exist, and prior to the injury this patient was functioning with a walker in her environment and independent in activities of daily living. The duration and frequency are acceptable and defended by objective data. Data not only describes numerically the wrist potential but also includes the prior functional levels to demonstrate the patient's potential to regain function with a course of therapy. This summary, as documented, has justified the need for therapy based on a strong therapy diagnosis of postoperative carpal tunnel and pain. The justification for the billing period is supported by the objective data, which show progress since the patient started treatment. The specific goals related to the plan justify the need for therapy to continue. Table 5–7 is a sample format that can be used in your clinic to prepare and/or review your monthly summary documentation.

MEDICARE DISCHARGE SUMMARY

When discharge of the patient to another setting is indicated or therapy is discontinued, a discharge summary must be written. The discharge summary resembles a monthly summary except that there is no recommendation made for why treatment should be continued in the current facility. However, the issues of why therapy and why therapy should be given during the claim period must be addressed. They must be addressed as follows:

1. Overall progress from the date of the evaluation as well as the progress in the last billing period should be described. This documented progress justifies both the current and the total billing period.
2. A plan of care that takes into consideration the potential need for future services should be included.

A discharge summary from one facility to another, should never state that all goals were met if the patient is being admitted for further therapy in a different environment. Rather, the statement should be that the facility's goals are met and indicate the need for further services either at a less intense level or in a different environment. If the therapist who discharges the patient indicates no further therapy in any setting is needed, there should be a statement of what the patient should continue to do on a home program or maintenance program. All therapists should remember the following:

1. The hospital therapist should be aware that a patient who is discharged to a skilled facility, primarily for further therapy, will need justification from the discharge summary that the patient is in need of further care but not in need of *intensive medical care*. A patient may be admitted to a skilled facility under Medicare *Part A* or *Part B*, depending on the intensity of the therapy the patient will be receiving.

2. The rehabilitation hospital patient who is discharged to another facility for further treatment should have unmet goals. The therapist receiving the patient should be aware that this patient has had a long course of therapy and should pay very specific attention to the unmet goals. Also, keep in mind that according to the Medicare regulations, the patient would not be a candidate for daily therapy because the intense therapy would warrant remaining in the rehabilitation hospital.

3. The skilled nursing facility therapist should keep in mind the alternative of home health services and include goals which address the need for assessment for the home environment.

In conclusion, a discharge summary does not mean that a patient is no longer in need of physical therapy. The summary should clearly state the future plan that is indicated for the patient, give an overview of the progress, and provide a projection of further needs of the patient. It is critical that the therapist plan for continuity of care through discharge summary. Table 9-5 which follows the case study can be used in your clinic to prepare and/or review your documentation

Case Study Discharge Summary

Read the following case study of a discharge summary (Table 5-8) as though you were a reviewer, determine if it includes documentation which justifies the therapy treatment, why there should be treatment during this billing period, and why treatment should be discontinued at this time.

TABLE 5–8.

DISCHARGE SUMMARY REPORT

Diagnosis: Open reduction, internal fixation of left hip This patient is receiving therapy for therapeutic exercises and gait training due to left hip fracture. The patient was authorized for non-weight-bearing gait training 2 weeks ago. Prior to that time, she was seen at bedside for passive and active assistive extremity strengthening exercises.	Why therapy?
Strength: The left lower extremity strength has improved from 2/5 to 3/5; left knee strength has improved from 3/5 to 3+/5. Right lower strength has improved from 3/5 to 3+/5 at the hip and from 3/5 to 3+/5 at the right knee. *Gait function:* Patient's gait has improved from requiring moderate to maximum assistance of three persons to ambulate non-weight-bearing on the left in the parallel bars, to ambulating one length in the parallel bars with minimal assistance of two persons on each side. A third person is needed to maintain the left lower extremity in a non-weight-bearing position. This patient is unable to be taught use of assistive device due to her inability to maintain non-weight-bearing stance on her own.	Why therapy continued
At this time, the patient has reached a plateau in her status. Since she will not be seen by the orthopedic physician for 1 month, she will be placed on a maintenance program. This program will maintain her present status with exercise and gait activities. Will plan to see this patient once again on a rehabilitation program when her weight-bearing status is changed by the physician. *Long-term goal:* Improve left lower extremity strength to 3+/5 and return to functional ambulation requiring minimal assistance of one person with an appropriate device.	Why discharged

Critiquing Discharge Summary

This discharge summary speaks to justification of therapy by noting the diagnosis of hip fracture. The progress note is written in objective terms and justifies the billing period. However, the summary does not present a strong justification for continuing therapy for this particular billing period. For that reason, the question arises as to why there was not an earlier discharge. Keeping in mind that the reviewer can only accept parts of the claim, this lack of justification jeopardizes full reimbursement. This situation could have been avoided if the therapist had written the progress note to include a description of the range and strength and functional changes from the time of the initial evaluation and those from the prior month. For example, the documentation could have read that "the left knee strength on evaluation was 2/5, last month 3−/5, and currently 3+/5." This specifically speaks to progress in both the current and the entire billing period. The reason for discharge is reasonable for the condition of the patient and also includes a future plan of care and indicates that therapy should be reinitiated. Clear, concise documentation assures that positive claims review will occur. It also allows all members of the health care team to gain an accurate understanding of the patient's problems so that there is a coordinated effort to establish a plan of care that will obtain maximum function levels for the patient. The major elements of a discharge summary are shown in Table 5–9; a sample format is shown in Table 5–10.

MEDICARE APPEAL PROCESS

Once a claim is submitted to the carrier or intermediary, it will be reviewed and a determination made to either pay or deny the claim. The main reasons for denial are that (1) the claim is for a noncovered service or (2) the claim is not considered reasonable and necessary.

A noncovered service is defined based on Medicare regulations, and there is no recourse for the provider. Claims for noncovered services are rarely seen by the reviewer. For example, a claim submitted with a diagnosis of fractured elbow with moist heat as the only treatment is not a covered service. Providing moist heat alone is not defined as skilled service according to the Medicare regulations. This type of claim should never be submitted, because it clearly is noncoverable.

On the other hand, if a claim is denied due to the determination that it was not "reasonable and necessary," the provider must decide whether to appeal the decision. Therapists should not ignore situations in which an appeal is appropriate. Reasons for appeal are (1) to defend the therapist's professional judgment, and (2) to have impact on future Medicare denials and appeals in formulation of the review guidelines for outpatient services

In the review process, both the therapist and the reviewer make judgment calls based on their individual interpretation of the Medicare regulations, and neither side is always correct. The denial should be appealed if the provider believes that (1) the therapy was necessary for the patient's condition, and (2) the goals were accomplished in a reasonable and timely fashion based on the Medicare regulation definitions.

TABLE 5–9.

ESSENTIAL ELEMENTS OF MEDICARE DISCHARGE SUMMARY

Diagnosis/reason for referral:	Why therapy?
Objective data: State overall impairment and function from the date of initial evaluation and last billing period to justify current and total billing period.	Why therapy continued?
Plan of care that takes into consideration need for future services. State only *goals met in your facility and that there is a need for further services at a less intense level or in a different environment.* If not appropriate, state what, if anything, the patient should continue to do on a home program or maintenance program.	Why discharged?

TABLE 5–10.

SAMPLE FORMAT FOR A MEDICARE DISCHARGE SUMMARY

	Why therapy?
	Why therapy continued?
	Why discharged?

Appeal Process for Medicare Part A

The appeal process for a Part A (inpatient service) is usually coordinated by the administrative personnel of the health care facility. The physical therapist may be involved only in submitting copies of all therapy documentation and a letter defending the claim. The Medicare regulation entitled "Billing Procedures" describes the specific process for appeal.

Appeal Process for Medicare Part B

The Part B (outpatient) appeal process is based on the section of the Medicare regulations entitled "Medical Review of Part B Bills and Billing Procedures." The therapist usually plays a major role in this process of appeal. Once again, the role of the physical therapist will be determined by the policy of the health care facility. The outpatient appeal process involves a great amount of paperwork, but once the provider has established a system to follow, the time involved is worth the potential outcome. In order to understand the appeal process, one must first understand the medical review process. There are two levels of medical review. They are described as Level I and Level II review.

Level I Review
Level I review evaluates claims based on

1. Facility and patient identification
2. Diagnosis
3. Duration
4. Number of visits
5. Date of onset
6. Date treatment was initiated
7. Billing period

If there is a problem with a claim at this level, the provider will receive notification requesting further information. The claim review at this level can not be based on *medical necessity*. If a notification for information is issued at this level, there usually has been a clerical error on the part of the provider. This can easily be corrected and the claim resubmitted for payment.

Level II Review
Level II review occurs if

1. The claim exceeds the limit set in the **edits,** which are listed in the Medicare regulation under the title of "Billing Procedures." The edits are a list of diagnoses which prescribe a set number of visits and duration in terms of months.
2. The diagnosis is not listed in the edits.
3. The intermediary who reviews the claim has chosen to review all submitted claims.
4. A focused medical review has occurred (the intermediary/carrier selects a focused category).

If the claim that has been reviewed at level II is denied, the provider and the beneficiary (patient) will receive a "Notice of Claim Determination." This notice will identify the period of the claim that is denied and the reason for the denial. The therapist or provider should review their documentation and determine if the claim should be appealed. The provider should request from the intermediary all documentation that pertains to the reviewer's decision to deny the claim. After review of these materials, the provider may request that the claim be reconsidered for payment. This may prompt the intermediary to request the full chart documentation from the provider. The provider may write a letter reviewing the claim and giving the rationale for submission of the claim. The content of the letter may not contain new information but must base the defense on the existing documentation. If the documentation is not concise and written according to Medicare standards, the provider may decide not to pursue appeal of the claim any further. If the appeal letter is submitted, the provider will receive in writing from the intermediary a second decision. If the claim is approved, payment will be made for the previously denied amount. If the claim is denied for the second time, the provider may request a hearing.

Hearing Process

There are three types of hearings involved in Medicare claims: in-person, telephone, or on-the-record hearings. The provider should notify the intermediary in writing as to the type of hearing being requested. The intermediary/carrier will notify the provider in writing regarding the date and time of the scheduled hearing.

A major concern of providers related to these hearing processes has been the questionable credentials of the hearing officers who conduct them. There is no specific job description or credentials for the position of a hearing officer. The individual may have received only on-the-job training and may have no medical background. Another concern is the potential that the hearing officer may consult with other personnel subsequent to the hearing in order to arrive at a decision. This practice is not permitted according to Medicare regulations. A fair hearing is one in which all parties have been involved in all discussion concerning the appealed claim and have had equal opportunity to defend their positions.

In-Person Hearing

If the choice is an in-person hearing, the provider may consider presenting expert witnesses, research articles, a history of payment, and any other information pertinent to the care of the patient to defend the claim. The complete chart and résumés of the witnesses who speak at the hearing should be submitted to the appeals officer. The determination of the appeal can only be based on the evidence presented at the hearing and from previous levels of the appeal process.

Telephone Hearing

If a provider chooses a telephone hearing, the therapist who treated the patient should be the individual involved in the appeal. If this individual is not available, the individual delegated to handle the appeal should be very familiar with the claim and with Medicare criteria for defending a "reasonable and necessary" claim.

On-the-Record Hearing

If the provider chooses an on-the-record hearing, all documentation should be resubmitted along with any other supportive material that defends the claim as reasonable and necessary. This type of appeal does not permit any verbal communication between the parties. This hearing is a request for review of the documentation once again. In summary, no matter what type of hearing is granted, the provider will be notified in writing regarding the decision of the hearing officer. The reason for the decision will be given and the specific section of the Medicare regulations on which the decision was based will be cited.

Administrative Law Judge Review

If the hearing process does not result in satisfactory resolution of the claim, the next level of appeal is the Administrative Law Judge Review. At this level, a provider should consider retaining legal counsel who is familiar with the Medicare appeal law. If the decision for denial is reversed at this level, payment for the claim will be made. If the decision of denial remains, the provider has no further level of appeal.

In summary, Medicare regulations delineate for the provider the rules for claims documentation. Because the decisions are based on individual interpretations of the criteria, there will always be room for disagreement in claims review. However, there are mechanisms in place, such as medical review and the appeal process, for both the provider and the intermediary/carrier to resolve differences. The provider needs to understand the Medicare regulations. The decision to treat or to accept the referral of a patient and submission of a claim to the Medicare program should be based on the therapist's professional judgment. The claim must be defended by documentation that demonstrates that the patient is eligible for coverage according to the Medicare definition of coverable services that are reasonable and necessary.

SUMMARY

Prior to initiating documentation, the Medicare regulations entitled "Coverage of Services and Billing Procedures" pertaining to the facility in which the service is being provided, should be read and thoroughly understood. A description of the two components of Medicare coverage (Part A and Part B) are contained in these documents. These documents will provide the therapist with a reference on which to determine a patient's eligibility for coverage under Medicare A or B (see Table 5–2). Once this determination has been made, documentation rules for Part A and Part B are basically the same.

Medicare documentation consists of an evaluation, a monthly summary, and a discharge summary. All documentation must use objective and measurable terminology. The documentation of a Medicare evaluation provides baseline data regarding the patient's condition and justifies the need for the physical therapist's skill to determine a reasonable and necessary plan of treatment for the patient. A Medicare monthly summary must address why therapy is indicated, why the patient was treated throughout the entire claims period, and why treatment should continue. The Medicare discharge summary is written when the decision is made to either discontinue therapy or discharge the patient to another facility for the remainder of the rehabilitation period. The discharge summary must not only show progress in the last billing period but also from the date of evaluation (see Table 5–9). The summary should contain a plan, keeping in mind the need for future services or a plan for maintenance or home program.

Complete and accurate documentation is vital for submission of a good claim. If the claim is not accepted for payment the Medicare regulations provide a process for appeal. The two main reasons for denial are noncovered services or a claim that is not considered to be reasonable and necessary. The claim should be appealed if the therapist believes that the therapy services were necessary for the patient's condition and that the goals were accomplished in a reasonable and timely fashion, based on definitions in the Medicare regulations. The Medicare Part A appeal is usually submitted by a facility's administration. The therapist may be involved only in submission of the therapy documentation. The Medicare regulation entitled "Billing Procedures" describes the specific process and should be read prior to submitting the appeal. The Medicare Part B appeal process is based on the regulation entitled "Medical Review of Part B Bills and Billing Procedures."

The three aspects of medical review are level I and level II reviews; in-person, telephone, and on-the-record hearings; and administrative law judge review.

This chapter has detailed the major criteria for which positive claims review under Medicare can be achieved. Examples have been provided for successful approval based on documented evidence that demonstrates justification of effective and reasonable and necessary services. Medicare reporting forms and excerpts from the Medicare manual relative to hospital, home health, skilled nursing, and the intermediary manual are included in Appendix III–A to G for your information.

Now that we have discussed the documentation requirements for Medicare reimbursement, test your knowledge of the various components. A sample case study with answers is presented at the end of this chapter along with a step-by-step review of the reports. Samples of report forms are included for you to use to review or practice Medicare report writing in your clinic.

REFERENCES

1. Medicare Hospital Manual, Transmittal 550, Publication 10, New Procedures—Effective date, November 11, 1988, Section 515, Billing for Part B, Outpatient Physical Therapy (OPT) Services, Washington, DC, 1988, Department of Health and Human Services, Health Care Financing Administration.
2. Medicare Skilled Nursing Facility Manual, Transmittal 262, Section 214, Publication 12, Covered Level of Care-General, Section 280.9, Custodial Care, Washington, DC, December 1987, Department of Health and Human Services, Health Care Financing Administration.
3. Medicare Skilled Nursing Facility Manual, Transmittal 270, Publication 12,

New Procedures—Effective date, November 11, 1988, Section 542, Billing for Part B, Outpatient Physical Therapy (OPT), Washington, DC, August 1988, Department of Health and Human Services, Health Care Financing Administration.

4. Medicare Intermediary Manual, Transmittal 1398, Section 3904, Publication 13-3, Part 3 Claims Process, New Procedures—Effective date, November 11, 1988, Medical Review (MR) of Part B, Intermediary Outpatient Physical Therapy (OPT) Bills, Washington, DC, 1988, Department of Health and Human Services, Health Care Financing Administration.

5. Plan of Care/Assessment for Outpatient Rehabilitation, Form HCFA-700, Washington, DC, Sept 1989, Department of Health and Human Services, Health Care Financing Administration.

6. Updated Plan of Care/Progress for Outpatient Rehabilitation, Form HCFA-701 (9/89), Washington, DC, 1989, Department of Health and Human Services, Health Care Financing Administration.

7. (Optional) Updated Progress for Outpatient Rehabilitation, Form HCFA-702 (9/89), Washington, DC, 1989, Department of Health and Human Services, Health Care Financing Administration.

TEST YOUR KNOWLEDGE

1. What is the simple definition of Medicare?
2. Who administers the Medicare program?
3. What is the difference between an intermediary and a carrier?
4. What are the two components of Medicare?
5. What is another term used to refer to Medicare Part A?
6. What is another term used to refer to Medicare Part B?
7. Where can a provider easily determine the patient's Medicare eligibility?
8. In what settings does Medicare Part A reimburse for physical therapy services?
9. In what settings does Medicare Part B reimburse for physical therapy services?
10. In what manual are Medicare regulations found?
11. The determination that qualifies a patient for admittance for Part A physical therapy coverage rather than Part B are based on what two criteria?
12. List the four criteria that define "reasonable and necessary" treatment.
13. What is the general purpose of an evaluation?
14. What three elements are included in an evaluation that determine justification for physical therapy intervention?
15. List the two methods used to determine the objective findings.
16. List the two types of goals that must be contained in Medicare documentation.
17. In a one-time evaluation or consultation, what must be documented instead of a plan and goals?
18. What three issues does a monthly summary address?
19. What two issues does a discharge summary address?
20. What are two reasons for denial of a Medicare claim?
21. What are the three levels of the Part B appeal process?
22. List the types of hearings in the Medicare Part B appeal process.

CASE STUDY

The case study is presented at the time of the initial referral for evaluation and again at the monthly summary. The first step in the process is to identify the problem or the reason for which the patient has been referred.

Once that problem is identified, never lose sight of it in your documentation. Your statement regarding the reason for referral assures that it is obvious to the intermediary reviewer that the professional judgment of the physical therapist is needed. Remember that there are three elements that must be included in the evaluation that are directed at justification for the physical therapy intervention. These are (1) the reason for referral, (2) the patient's pertinent medical history, and (3) the level of previous and current function.

Case Study at Initial Evaluation

This 70-year-old woman who was hospitalized because of a flare-up of rheumatoid arthritis was recently discharged to home. Prior to the hospital admission, the patient was independent in her home with the aid of a quad cane and was able to manage activities of daily living in her small apartment. This woman lives alone, and is alert, well-oriented, and has a cooperative, pleasant nature. Her major complaint is that because of knee pain she is unable to walk or get around by herself.

Evaluation reveals that she has full range of motion in her upper extremities except for her right shoulder, which is limited to 110 degree rotation because of a previously fractured humerus. There are obvious arthritic changes in her knees. Because she is in pain you are unable to accurately measure knee range of motion. However, she does exhibit incomplete extension of both knees. Muscle testing of all extremities reveals that she has normal strength within functional limits and for her age. When the patient is asked to move her upper extremities you are able to discern a pain level ratio of 8/10 in both extremities. However, the lower extremities on the patient's attempt at ambulation is 9/10, especially in the knees, with the right knee being the most painful. To assess her ability to ambulate with a walker, moderate assistance of two people was required, and the patient ambulated 30 ft. During all attempts at ambulation the patient complained of severe pain in her right knee.

A sample Medicare Initial Evaluation Documentation Form is presented in Table 5–11, so that you can practice documentation and clinical reasoning skills. (Table 5–13, in the answer section of this chapter, illustrates the correct documentation of the initial evaluation of this case study.) When preparing your report, consider the answers to the following questions: What goals should be set for this patient in the initial evaluation? How could you set a rationale that the treatment intervention was appropriate for physical therapy and that the treatment intervention needs the expertise of a physical therapist? Based on the evaluation, are the goals and treatment plan rea-

TABLE 5–11.

Sample Format for Initial Evaluation

S:	Justification for referral
O:	Pertinent medical history
A:	Prior level of function
	Assessment of findings
P:	Treatment plan and goals

sonable and necessary for this patient's reason for referral? Have you considered the following in your documentation?

Reason for referral:

1. Included a list of diagnoses.
2. Reviewed the diagnosis list and determined the therapy diagnosis or reason for the evaluation.
3. Listed the pertinent medical history.
4. Stated prior level of function.
5. Reviewed the objective findings and expanded on them in documentation, for example:
   a. Range of motion in ratio form.
   b. Detailed description of the knee pain.
   c. Description of transfer in terms of assistance, equipment needs, and how intervention will improve overall function.
   d. Description of gait in terms of assistance, device, patient technique (e.g., steppage, speed, posture, space of base).
6. Reviewed your goals to make sure they:
   a. State the baseline findings and show a comparison between the baseline and anticipated gains.
   b. Are written so that they are measurable and functional.
7. Your plan is concise and demonstrates that:
   a. The duration of treatment is necessary and reasonable for the diagnosis.
   b. The appropriate modality with anticipated outcome has been made and is the best alternative available for the condition being treated.
   c. The type of therapeutic exercise selected is appropriate for the patient's condition.
   d. A rationale for concentration on specific joints is clearly stated.
   e. Gait training will result in progression to another device.

The next step in the process is to report on the patient's progress, to justify why the patient was treated throughout the claim period, and to recommend further treatment or discharge.

CASE STUDY FOR MONTHLY SUMMARY/DISCHARGE SUMMARY

After 2 weeks of treatment the patient indicates to you that she is doing much better. She can walk again without a lot of pain. She has been receiving treatment three times a week for 2 weeks. The therapy consisted of moist heat to the knees bilaterally followed by 20 minutes of ultrasound at 1.5

WPC2. The program included active and active resistive exercise to knees, followed by gait training. The patient's chief complaint on evaluation was that an acute episode of pain due to a flare-up of rheumatoid arthritis had caused her to be hospitalized for 1 week. After discharge she was unable to ambulate with a walker in her living environment. With the above treatment the pateint has made the following progress: Her strength has increased bilaterally from 3/4 to 4/4. Her pain level has decreased from 9/10 to 0−3/10 during active motion and 8/10−0/10 at rest. The edema and redness of the right knee are no longer present. She has progressed to independent ambulation with the walker. How would you answer the Key Questions regarding Medicare: Why therapy? Why treated throughout the period of the claim? Why should therapy be continued or why should the patient be discharged?

Table 5−12 is provided so you can practice writing a Monthly Summary or Discharge Summary based on the new information. The report should be written with the idea of outpatient referral. (A sample report format for this summary report appears in Table 5−14 in the answer section of this chapter.) When writing your Monthly Summary or Discharge Summary report, have you considered the following important aspects of the report?

1. Why therapy was indicated.
2. Why therapy was needed for the whole billing period.
3. Why therapy was discontinued and whether it was reasonable to do so.
4. Whether there is a future plan.
5. Are the four criteria for "reasonable and necessary" met in the content of the documentation?
    a. Is treatment accepted medical practice for the patient's condition?
    b. Is the service of the complexity and sophistication that only a physical therapist can perform the treatment?
    c. Is there an expectation that the condition will improve significantly in a reasonable and predictable time frame?
    d. Are the amount, frequency, and duration of treatment reasonable?

TABLE 5–12.

Sample Format for Discharge Summary

	Why therapy?
	Why therapy continued?
	Why discharged?

TEST YOUR KNOWLEDGE ANSWER SHEET

1. Federal health insurance.
2. Health Care Financing Administration (HCFA).
3. An intermediary is an insurance entity response for claims submitted on behalf of a client by a hospital, skilled nursing facility, home health agency, hospice, and other providers of services. A carrier is responsible for claims submitted on behalf of a client by the physician or other health care providers.
4. Medicare Part A and Medicare Part B.
5. Hospital insurance.
6. Medical insurance.
7. Medicare insurance card.
8. Inpatient hospital, inpatient skilled nursing facility, and home health agency.
9. Outpatient hospital, skilled nursing facility, home health agency, CORF rehabilitation facility, and private practice office.
10. *Health Insurance Manual.*
11. Need for daily therapy and intensity of therapy.
12. a. The therapy is of a level of complexity and sophistication that only a physical therapist can render the service.
    b. The therapy is accepted medical practice for the condition.
    c. There must be an expectation that the therapy will cause the condition to significantly improve in a reasonable and predictable period of time.
    d. The amount, frequency, and duration of the therapy are reasonable.
13. An evaluation documents a baseline on the patient's condition.
14. a. Reason for referral.
    b. Pertinent medical history.
    c. Patient's previous level of function.
15. a. Tests and measurements.
    b. Functional loss.
16. a. Measurable.
    b. Functional.
17. The therapist must make recommendations, teach the patient, or initiate changes in the patient's program.
18. a. Why therapy is needed.
    b. Why there is justification for treatment during the claim period.
    c. Why therapy needs to continue.
19. a. Overall progress and specific progress of the last claim period.
    b. Plan for future services.

20. a. Noncovered service.
    b. Services are not reasonable and necessary.
21. a. Levels I and II reviews.
    b. Hearings.
    c. Administrative law judge.
22. a. In-person hearing.
    b. Telephone hearing.
    c. On-the-record hearing.

TABLE 5–13.

MEDICARE INITIAL EVALUATION

Diagnosis: Gait dysfunction, pain secondary to rheumatoid arthritis

S: Patient states, "My pain is terrible. I can't use my knees."	Justification for referral
O: Right knee flexion is 55/90 with extension lag of 20. Left knee flexion is 90/90 with extension lag of 15. The right knee displays hot, reddened area over medial aspect. The knee is painful to touch, and the pain increases with flexion of the joint. There is moderate edema. Patient states pain is most severe when standing.	
Transfer: Patient needs minimal assistance of one to move from supine to sitting position. Assistance is needed to move the lower right extremity. To move from sit to stand, the patient needs moderate assistance of one to stand with the walker.	Pertinent medical history
Pain: On active movement of upper extremities, patient's pain is 8/10. Lower extremities display pain upon ambulation. Pain is 9/10 in both knees.	
Ambulation: Patient is able to ambulate with walker and moderate assistance of two for approximately 30 ft. During ambulation, patient knees flexed and takes small shuffling steps. She needs assistance to move walker because of fear of increased pain in right knee on stepping. The increased pain during ambulation prevents patient from using proper steppage with walker; therefore, gait is not safe.	
Prior to flare-up of arthritis, patient was independent with cane in living environment.	Prior level of function
A: Increased pain during ambulation prevents patient from ambulating safely. With decrease in pain patient should be able to return to previous living arrangement. She will be able to use the quad cane safely to perform ADLs.	Assessment of findings
P: Decrease pain from 9/10 to 0/10 in right knee. Improve gait from moderate assist of two with walker to independent ambulation with walker and progress to quad cane.	
Treat 3 times per week for 2 weeks. Moist heat to right knee followed by ultrasound, active and isometric exercise to right knee, and active and active resistive exercise to left knee. Gait training with walker.	Treatment plan and goals

TABLE 5–14.

Diagnosis: Acute pain, gait dysfunction	
S: Patient states, "I am doing much better. I can walk again without a lot of pain."	Why therapy?
O: Patient has been receiving physical therapy three times per week for 2 weeks. Therapy has consisted of moist heat to knees bilaterally, followed by 20 minutes of ultrasound therapy at 1.5 WPC2; active and active-resistive exercises to knees; and gait training. The patient's chief complaint was an acute episode of pain due to flare-up of rheumatoid arthritis, followed by hospitalization for 1 week. Pain altered her ability to ambulate independently with a walker in her living environment.	
Pain: Evaluation revealed a normal left knee and edema throughout the right knee. The patient had complained that pain increased on ambulation, particularly in the right knee. The pain was graded at 9/10 on ambulation, and 7/10 on rest. Strength was 3/4 in knee flexion bilaterally, and both knees lacked 25 degrees of full extension. Therapist administered moist heat and ultrasound to the patient's knees and noted the following progress: Decrease in pain from 9/10 to 0–3/10 during active motion and 8/10 to 0/10 during rest. Edema and redness of right knee no longer present.	
Strength: Therapy, which included active and active-resistive exercise to the knees, accomplished the following: Strength increased from 3/4 to 4/4 bilaterally. Patient progressed to independent ambulation with walker due to increases in strength in the right knee.	Why treated throughout period of claim?
Gait: Gait training was responsible for returning patient to previous level of independent ambulation with walker. On evaluation the patient was unable to ambulate farther than 5 ft with moderate assistance of two persons and with a walker. The gait was slow, shuffling, and not safe. Patient was taught in parallel bars to take equal steps, to toe off and heel strike, and to use the musculature of the knees and feet to allow the feet to clear the floor. The patient was instructed in a three-point gait, using the walker to give right knee support.	

(Continued.)

TABLE 5–14 (cont.).

Diagnosis: Acute pain, gait dysfunction	
A: With decreased pain, increased strength in knees, and teaching gait technique, patient was able to progress from ambulation with a walker and moderate assistance of two, a distance of 5 ft to independent ambulation with a walker. The patient was able to ambulate with a safe gait that allowed her an active and independent role in her activities of daily living. The therapy made it possible for the patient to return to prior level of function.	
P: Therapy is being discontinued at this time. Patient has been instructed in proper application of a home moist heat unit and an exercise program for her knees. She has been given written instructions. Patient is to continue to do exercises and apply heat for 2 more weeks, then call the therapist.	Why therapy continued or why patient discharged?

CHAPTER 6

Quality Assurance and Total Quality Management

Corinne T. Ellingham, M.S., PT

Susan H. Abeln, PT, A.R.M.

Key Concepts

- Quality care
- Position of the profession on quality assurance
- Five-step process for incorporating quality improvement

QUALITY CARE

Questions Reflecting Definitions of Quality

Quality is often defined in terms of "the degree of excellence" that a thing possesses.[1] This meaning of quality is generally agreed upon. Yet, at one time, health care professionals thought it was not necessary to define, measure, or explore the quality of the U.S. health care system because a quality of service was always assumed to exist. Payers often felt that way also. In the past, "the health care system was a black box with trusted physicians (and other practitioners) inside doing, payers assumed, the right thing."[2] However, with the passage of time, the changes in the health care system discussed in Chapter 1 have changed these assumptions. Now many practitioners are involved in quality assurance. They assess the quality of patient care by considering whether the care provided and the documentation of that care met standards they have set. In their opinion, a patient receives quality care when that care meets some or all of the following criteria:

1. Is provided by a clinician who has participated routinely or in professional development experiences
2. Generates therapist or staff satisfaction
3. Is consistently provided by the same therapist or practitioner
4. Meets the standard of care in their community/region or nation

This list mirrors what professionals now believe to be key determinants or elements of quality care (Table 6–1). However, none of these standards consider how the patient perceives this care. A deeper look at quality care is obviously needed. Does the care guarantee that patients are satisfied with their treatment? Do the patients believe they have received good or "quality" care? Would the patient return to the therapist who provided the service? Were they treated as "individuals" rather than "cases"? In other words, did the care provided and the documentation of that care demonstrate that the care

- Generated patient satisfaction
- Provided symptomatic relief to the patient

TABLE 6–1.

HIGH-PRIORITY DETERMINANTS OR ELEMENTS OF QUALITY CARE (MODIFIED FOR CLARITY)*

Professionals perceive quality when they
   Can practice current state of the profession
   Have autonomy
   Can provide the patient with optimal care
Consumers perceive quality when practitioners
   Quickly recognize the consumers' perceived
     needs
   Are courteous and communicate concern
Consumers perceive quality when they (the
   consumers)
   Get better with care provided
   Are able to function and return to vocation and
     avocation
Third-party payers perceive quality when it is
   demonstrated that there is
   Efficient, effective use of funds
   Client satisfaction
   Client return to work/functional level

*Modified from Roberts JS, Prevost JA: *The Internist: Health Policy in Practice*, Washington, DC, American Society for Internal Medicine, Sept 1987, p 11.

- Met or exceeded patient expectations for the treatment
- Added to the general well being of the patient

These factors are a partial listing of critical elements of quality care according to patients who are the consumers of health care (see Table 6–1).

However, meeting all of these standards does not guarantee that the patients are getting well or that they are even improving. Perhaps further quality checks should be added which look at whether the care has

- Effected complete resolution of the objective findings
- Led to an improved clinical outcome
- Led to a quantifiable functional improvement
- Generally improved the health status of the patient

We believe these sets of quality checks must be added to address quality care as defined by another key constituency: the payer. It creates personal satisfaction for the physical therapist when the expectations of both the providers and the patients are met related to quality care, but we must recognize that, for most current practitioners, much of the revenue from one's practice does not come from your patient's pocket. Most of your income is from other payer sources. Therefore, it is important that the payers and employers are satisfied. To them, quality care is evident when the care meets some or all of the following criteria:

1. Is appropriately and completely documented
2. Leads to quantifiable functional improvement within the limits of reimbursement
3. Lowers the total work days lost due to an injury or illness
4. Makes the maximum possible contribution to the reduction of lost productivity
5. Is cost-effective (see Table 6–1; Fig 6–1)

Few providers today would disagree that all these elements need to be addressed in the standard established for their practice. As physical therapists we must address most or all of these elements to assess and ensure the quality of care in our practice.

Other Ways to Look at Quality Care

By now, it should be obvious that a dictionary definition of quality as "the degree of excellence" a thing possesses is not much help in defining

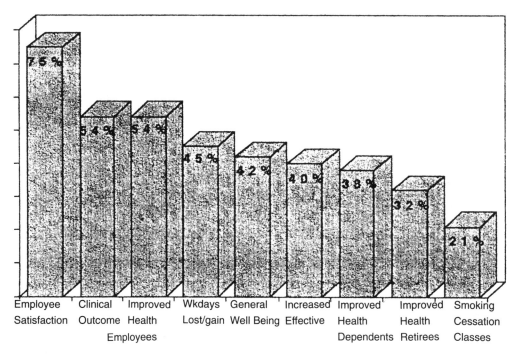

FIG 6–1.
Corporate views on health care quality. Which factors are "very important" in evaluating health care quality?

quality in health care. Deciding what is quality of care often depends on who you are. Prior to attempting to discuss techniques and methodologies to assure or measure quality, we are still left with the question, "What is quality care? The Institute of Medicine definition of quality, as reported to Congress in May of 1990, ties together two of the critical factors. They define quality as, "The degree to which health services for individuals and populations increase the likelihood of the *desired outcome* and are consistent with the current professional knowledge."[3] Leaders in the physical therapy profession have built on this definition. They proposed that quality is *the effect of our actions* on the overall satisfaction and well being of those to whom we provide services. If you accept this proposition, you might agree that quality means being:

- Effective in improving health and/or ability to function
- Valued for our services
- Supportive of continuous efforts to improve quality
- Responsible for competence of staff
- Cost effective

- Assured patients are satisfied with the accuracy, timeliness, efficiency, thoroughness, availability, and courtesy of our services

These same leaders further proposed that quality means achieving the outcomes and goals expected by payers, employers, patients, utilization review firms, and others as well as those expected by the patients. These disparate parties have differing views regarding what they consider to be quality care. Many are primarily concerned with the use of funds for efficient, effective treatment and that their clients are able to return to work or previous functional level. Providers, in their attempts to demonstrate that the care provided is effective and efficient, have been "embarrassed to realize how little it does is of known, scientifically proven, efficacy; perhaps less than 20% of what physicians do every day has been shown to be of clear value in well designed clinical studies."[2] Because of these efficacy studies and initial research on the variation in practice patterns, the payers' pessimism and even ire concerning the quality of health care has been raised. Payers no longer assume that physicians and other practitioners are doing the right thing or that high-quality patient care exists. Indeed, payers are perhaps the principal driving force in the quest for quality health care. They, along with a number of health care policy makers and a few medical professionals, have begun to more completely explore the characteristics of quality care and of variation in practice patterns by providers. The payers have undertaken this effort in order to understand what kind of care they are paying so much money to provide to their health care policy holders and how that care compares with "quality care." They are aggressively seeking ways to control the costs of the care received, principally through control of variation in practice. Further, they are promoting research "to help them define standards for (quality) care, review procedures and quality measurement systems."[2] In other words, they are trying to specify "quality care" and then control any perceived variation by an individual provider away from any quality standards they develop. Their efforts are just beginning to reach critical mass now.

Four Pillars of Quality

Four distinct areas for current and future quality care research have evolved within the past decade. Donald Berwick, M.D., of the Harvard Community Health Plan (HCHP), one of the leaders in the use of the industry's quality improvement methods in health care, proposes that these four areas represent the intellectual pillars needed to support all future efforts on quality.[2] Some say they also form the foundation for a more complete definition of quality care, and that therefore, these four areas *must* be pursued.[2] These critical areas are

1. *Efficacy* of care practices (knowing what works)
2. *Appropriateness* of decisions (doing what works)
3. *Execution* of care (doing well what works)
4. *Purpose* of care (clarifying the values that tell us what we wish to do)[2] The information in Table 6–2 expands Table 6–1 to include elements of these four key areas (the key determinants of quality from major segments of the population) within it and in Figure 6–1.

Examination of each of these four key areas provides a better understanding of quality and its dimensions before we proceed to discuss mechanisms to assure it or manage it.

Efficacy: Knowing What Works

To practice quality care, a provider must know the efficacy of both the specific intervention or treatment approach and total components of the course of care. In medicine, the Office of Health Technology Assessment estimates that effectiveness has been shown by randomized[2] clinical trial for fewer than 20% of common medical practices. Only two of 26 new medical technologies currently under review for possible reimbursement have been subjected to randomized trials. An earlier review by Williamson and co-workers in 1986 looked at the scientific soundness of the information that

TABLE 6–2.

HIGH-PRIORITY ELEMENTS OF QUALITY IN HEALTH CARE*

Professionals perceive quality when they
   Can practice current state of the profession (efficacy, appropriateness, execution of care)
   Have autonomy (purpose)
   Can provide the patient with optimal care (efficacy, appropriateness, execution of care, purpose)
Consumers perceive quality when practitioners
   Quickly recognize consumers' perceived needs (execution of care, appropriateness)
   Are courteous and communicate concern (execution of care)
Consumers perceive quality when consumers
   Get better with care provided (efficacy, appropriateness)
   Are able to function and return to vocation/avocation (efficacy, appropriateness)
Third-party payers perceive quality when it is demonstrated that there is
   Efficient, effective use of funds (efficacy, appropriateness, purpose)
   Client satisfaction (execution of care)
   Clients return to work/functional level (efficacy, appropriateness, execution of care)

*Modified From Roberts JS, Prevost JA: *The Internist: Health Policy in Practice*, Sept 1987, p 11.

---

reaches the practitioners.[4] This study indicated that fewer than 10% of the evaluated research publications meet generally acceptable criteria for producing usable numbers. Many physical therapy treatments and procedures also have been shown to be minimally effective and inadequately researched. This lack of knowledge of the efficacy of health care and physical therapy practices is hard for some physical therapists to admit and even harder for patients and the payers to accept. Whose job is it to generate data or information stating what works and what does not work in health care? Should the federal government through its research arm, the major professional organizations, and the leading scientific organizations have the responsibility for assessing the efficacy of various health care practices? No matter which organization is ultimately responsible, this does not mean that individual practitioners have no responsibility. They *must* cooperate with broad-based data collection efforts and participate in studies of efficacy when asked, and also conduct and disseminate single-subject research of their own as often as possible.

Appropriateness: Doing What Works

Reviews of quality cannot wait until all the research on efficacy has been completed. Therefore, a great deal of attention is currently being focused on improving the decision making process in patient care. *Improved decision making* studies generally favor highly structured methods and endorse *explicit estimation* over **implicit judgment.** Using this approach, many have begun to develop **community standards, guidelines,** or **algorithms of care.** For example, the HCHP has developed more than 30 algorithms for the care of common ambulatory conditions. Each algorithm was developed by a team of suitably constituted experts within HCHP. They reviewed all pertinent, available information (including existing efficacy studies) and through a nominal group process agreed on an algorithm for care for a particular condition. An effort was made to keep the algorithm as close as possible to the practice environment of the practitioners who would be using them. The Society for Medical Decision Making is also very involved in promoting and developing clinical decision making. Their efforts are directed toward the development of guidelines. The sequence of steps they followed to develop guidelines is seen in Table 6–3.

The same kind of process has also been done by physical therapists in Minnesota. Over a period of several years, the Minnesota Chapter of the American Physical Therapy Association convened several panels of experts who reviewed all existing literature and opinion concerning specific conditions, and developed community standards for care of a limited number of diagnoses. These standards were presented to physical therapists across the

TABLE 6–3.

STEPS FOR THE DEVELOPMENT OF GUIDELINES BY EXPERT PANELS*

1. Choose a clinical condition from the priorities based on prevalence, morbidity/mortality, potential for benefit, variability in practice, high costs of treatment, and importance to Medicare beneficiaries and other populations of public health importance.
2. Clearly define the clinical condition or treatment to be considered for the development of a guideline and its intended users.
3. Review and analyze the literature and available scientific evidence of appropriateness and effectiveness.
4. Review the estimates of outcomes important to patients that will be influenced by intervention.
5. Review the benefits and harms from use of each intervention.
6. Review health outcomes and costs generated by the intervention.
7. Conduct open forums to provide an opportunity to groups and individuals to present information and comments.
8. Prepare the first draft of the guideline.
9. Revise draft guidelines after analysis of guideline pretesting and of comments from external peer review.
10. Prepare and disseminate guideline in appropriate forms for use by providers, consumers, and educators.
11. Evaluate assimilation of the guideline into clinical practice and revise as indicated.

*From McCormick KA: Presented at Forum for Quality and Effectiveness in Health Care. Society for Medical Decision Making. Used by permission.

state for feedback. After all comments were in and revision had occurred, they were used as educational tools for the professional community and the payers within the state. These community standards as well as algorithms and guidelines are, in Berwick's opinion "a convenient way to convey existing scientific data into action. When scientific data are lacking, they can be conscientious best guesses [and therefore] are better than the random variation" of practice.[2] Guidelines or algorithms are usually developed to reduce variation from practice to practice; to reduce uncertainty about quality, efficacy, and effectiveness; and to reformat existing information that could improve clinical decision making but is not now in an easily usable format.[5] The development of algorithms by the Harvard group and of community standards by the Minnesota physical therapists have led to a flood of requests for copies of these documents from major corporations, insurance companies, and other payers. While payers desperately want this kind of material, often we practitioners fear it. This may be because we have been taught to fear "cookbook" medicine and fear the loss of our autonomy in clinical decision making. We must move past these fears. Algorithms and/or guidelines simply specify appropriate care based on research, expert judgement, and practice environment. They allow us to provide better health care by facilitating scientific review. It is the opinion of most experts that algorithms or other similar guidelines and protocols will soon be a widespread fact of life for every health care provider. If this is so, we believe that leadership for their development should come from within our profession. We must proclaim loudly and clearly acceptable and preferred patterns of practice. We *must* oppose thoughtless, ineffective, and inefficient practices that lead to too much or too little care. We must not only speak strongly for doing what works but also demonstrate by our actions that we *do* what works; we do it well, and, in fact, we do it better than others!

Execution: Doing Well That Which Works

Knowing what works and doing what works do not guarantee that we will provide better quality health care to patients or achieve better outcomes. We must be certain that in our day-to-day efforts we maintain consistently high standards of quality in the way we do the things that work. We need to avoid falling below these standards because of inherent defects in our complex medical system, excessive waste in our work practices, unjustified complexity built into our practices over the course of time, or wide frequent unpredictable variations from our intended aims.

How can we be assured that we are maintaining high standards of quality? Perhaps by learning the lesson the Japanese learned after World War II, when they transformed their industrial practices by paying heed to the work of modern American quality experts like W. Edwards Deming, Joseph Juran, and Philip B. Crosby, all of whom promoted quality and its continuous improvement. Can similar quality improvement techniques be applied to health care? Several medical organizations believe the answer is *yes* and have taken major steps in implementing these methods. Notable in this group are Hospital Corporation of America in many of its hospitals; EPIC Healthcare Group of Dallas; the Harvard Community Health Plan in Massachusetts; Meritor Hospital in Madison, Wisconsin; and the Henry Ford Health System in Detroit. The Deming, Juran, and Crosby techniques ask us to study the *processes* by which patients receive specific care. Their techniques ask us to look at those processes for sources of hazard, deficiency, defect, or time delay. They focus on making each process more statistically stable by reducing variability. Processes are examined for two distinct types of variations: *common cause variation*, which always occur as a part of the process (such as temperature variation in a non-climate-controlled treatment room); and *special cause variation*, which results from something unexpected happening (for example, an earthquake destroys your New York clinic and you have no place to treat patients or equipment to treatment them with). First, any special cause variations are eliminated (for example, fix a situation that could never have been expected—always prepare a backup treatment site and arrange for use of alternative minimal equipment); then the process is modified and/or improved to eliminate the common cause variation (for example, reassess and modify the process that leads to this problem through a variety of critical process analyses). The result is higher quality health care and consistently better outcome.

Purpose: Knowing What Is Right

A few experts have proposed that perhaps the greatest challenge to be faced in improving the quality of health care is the need to "regain focus on what exactly health care as a social enterprise exists to accomplish."[2] This, in turn, raises a potentially more relevant question: "To what extent is health care a *social good?*" A "social good," as economists use the term, implies a commodity or service paid for in such a way that the user, after consumption, is *economically whole;* that is, the user is as wealthy after consuming the good as before."[2] To address "social goodness" forces us to look at the value of health care. As discussed in Chapter 1, the economics of health care is concerned with "ensuring that society gets the best return possible in terms of human welfare from the resources available."[5] We must determine what quality of life (as a result of medical care) society can expect from us. This question has no easy answer, but to provide quality care we believe that each of us, as a resource in the health care delivery system, must examine our practices to see if we are helping or hindering *society as a whole* (not an individual patient) to obtain the maximum good from us. To illustrate this point, let us look at a real case depicting a physical therapist who has to daily consider if society is getting the best return possible in terms of human welfare. Even though this situation did not occur within the United States, it is applicable to every environment. Let us travel to the northwest corner of Australia to a region as large as Great Britain. Because of the region's sparse population, one physical therapist, Jill, was given the responsibility by the provincial government of providing physical therapy care for the region. The programs she developed *had* to be designed to maximize the good from her services to the entire region. Consequently, she created a program based on outreach and education. Jill chose to provide no-hands-on care because she believed that by allocating her limited resources, her time, and her expertise to the intensive care of even one individual she would be negatively impacting the health of the entire region. Although this case is an extreme, as time advances and the resources within the health care system decrease steadily, we believe all therapists should consider their role in maximizing the health of their "designated region."

In summary, we have delved into numerous definitions and aspects of quality care. We recognize that each of us has different values and expectations for quality care. So what is the best definition of quality? We do not believe that there is a "best" definition. We suggest, however, that to develop a good working quality care standard for practice, one must look carefully at each of the parties who has a stake in the care of your patients: the patient, the provider, the referral source, the employer (who provides the medical benefits), the payer, the claims adjuster, and so forth. Any definition of quality care should include the critical elements for quality care from each stakeholders' viewpoint, and must also incorporate Berwick's four elements—*efficacy* (knowing what works); *appropriateness* (using what works); *execution* (doing well that which works); and *purpose* (clarifying the values that tell us what we wish to do.)—into a practice's model standard of quality care.

Small qa Moves to Large QA

Let us move on to look at methods that have been used or can be used to ensure that quality care exists in our practices. Early methods to assure quality in health care usually focused on punishment. Physicians in ancient Mesopotamia, for example, lost a body part (e.g., a hand or an eye) each time their treatment caused a patient harm. While quality assurance methods have changed greatly over the years, most have continued to focus on sanctions, if not direct punishment, rather than on improvement in care. Cited as evidence of this point of view are the overemphasis on the clinical aspects of care, compartmentalization of quality assurance activities, overattention to the performance of individuals ("bad apples") and the lack of attention to the processes through which patient care is delivered.[4] When it finally was recognized that *quality can never be assured but rather at best only be improved*,[4] the movement from quality assurance to quality improvement began. One of the more popular current approaches is Total Quality Management (TQM), which is based on the concept of continuous quality improvement.[7] A TQM approach provides a wide variety of methods for health care professionals to utilize in their efforts in striving for quality. J.W. Williamson's framework for measuring and improving quality outcomes includes both traditional and emerging systems and refers to them both as *quality management* (QM). As early as 1970, de Gyndt[8] identified the five critical functional areas he felt should be used in measuring quality within health care:

- **Structure:** Measurement of qualifications of staff, physical structure, licensure, professional credentials
- **Process:** Measurement of what a health care practitioner does
- **Outcome:** Measurement of a patient's outcome

- **Content:** Measurement of appropriateness of care (utilization)
- **Impact:** Measurement of the impact of care on society

Because Williamson et al.[7] believe that QM is "a continuous function to systematically assess and improve health care as a whole or any of its specific clinical, administrative, or support functions," they agree that each of these areas are important for consideration. Also pertinent are these following thoughts on quality and outcomes related to their QM approach. Their beliefs mirror those of Berwick, that is, that the purpose of quality improvement is improved outcomes and that "Outcomes can be defined as results of any health care process, involving either the consumer or provider of care, and measured at any specified point in time. There can be health, economic, or societal outcomes. For example, health outcomes can be measured in quality of life for either the patient or the provider. Economic outcomes can be measured in monetary terms related to patient earning loss averted or provider care costs saved. Societal outcomes are less tangible and include factors such as satisfaction, education, ethical-legal, or even religious results of care, again involving either the consumer or the provider."[7]

The basis of this framework for Williamson et al. is the move from small qa (quality assurance) to LARGE QA (quality improvement). The approaches they label as small qa require *inductive* reasoning. These "focus on structure and process and assume (or induce) that improved outcomes will result if these are changed." An example of this approach would be the requirement of mandatory continuing education in order to achieve relicensure. Legislators and therapists who recommend such laws make an inductive judgement which assumes that a physical therapist attending continuing education courses and workshops will gain knowledge (structure) that will improve the patient care (process) and, ultimately, patient health (outcomes). A further example of small qa thinking is evident in the first set of practitioner quality standards referred to earlier. When care is provided by a clinician who has participated routinely in professional development experiences; or when it generates therapist or staff satisfaction; or when it is consistently provided by the same therapist or practitioner; or when it meets the standard of care in the community, region, or nation, an inductive leap to a conclusion is still required to assume that this will ensure a high level of professional knowledge (structure) that will improve patient care (process) and patient health (outcomes). Approaches that Williamson and colleagues label as LARGE QA approaches are based on *deductive* reasoning. These generally begin with an unacceptable or less than optimal outcome and identify structures or processes that should be changed to improve that specific outcome. An example of LARGE QA would focus on a specific outcome, such as the failure to return to work of 30% of the patients in one clinic's work hardening program, and then *deductively identify* those structures (several therapists administering treatment have not had any training in work hardening) or processes (the clinic did not attempt to ascertain from any source the true functional job demands of the injured employee's position nor communicate with the employer at any time) whose change might result in measureable improvement impact. The scope of small qa, Williamson's group states, "is narrow, focusing on variables easily measured," such as isolated facts in written board examinations. LARGE QA is seen as more comprehensive. It seeks evidence that a solution to the problem exists, and ultimately examines ways to substantially improve the situation. Its central emphasis is on outcome. Whereas small qa assures society of minimum competence, LARGE QA offers promises of higher levels of effectiveness, better outcomes, and excellence.[7] Characteristics of small qa and LARGE QA are compared in Table 6–4.

Williamson and co-workers recognize the importance of both types of quality management approaches but strongly advocate that a major emphasis be placed on LARGE QA activities. They suggest that the first step a provider must take to develop this LARGE QA approach is to develop an orientation to outcomes. This orientation demonstrates an understanding that the "product of health care needs to be defined as 'benefits achieved', *not* 'units of services'; and these benefits MUST be defined in terms of outcomes, *not* improved processes or structures."[7] The outcomes to which they refer relate directly to their earlier definition of positive outcomes (one that improves either the health, economic, or societal outcomes). These researchers state that the purpose of any quality management technique is to identify

TABLE 6–4.

COMPARISON OF SMALL qa AND LARGE **QA**

Small qa (Quality Assurance)	Large QA (Quality Improvement)
Program	Process
Coordinator/Director, Committee driven	Management driven
No historical value for customer input	Consumer driven
Assign responsibility for monitoring	Organize knowledgeable team
Delineate scope of care and identify most important aspects of care	Find a process improvement opportunity
Systematic monitoring based on indicators	Clarify current knowledge of process
Establish thresholds focus on special causes	Strive for continuous improvement, reduce variation
Monitor care by collecting and organizing data for each indicator	Uncover root causes of variation
Evaluate care when thresholds indicates: Improve Care Identify Problem	Start improvement cycle

and maximize what they call "achievable benefits not achieved" (ABNA). An example of this is shown in Figure 6–2. In this figure, the vertical scale depicts health states; the horizontal scale represents time. The three graphic lines depict the changing health status of an imagined patient for three different suppositions:

- Progression of disability if no formal medical care
- Progression of disability with care currently received
- Progression of disability under optimal conditions of care

Area A represents health benefits achieved; and *Area B* represents ABNA, which Williamson et al.[7] state is the main focus of LARGE QA quality management approaches. This construct can be used for other measurable health care outcomes such as patient satisfaction or for monitoring tort claims. Its most important use is in establishing priorities for quality management activities. If a topic has a great opportunity for improvement (a large ABNA), they propose that it should be given the highest priority for study.

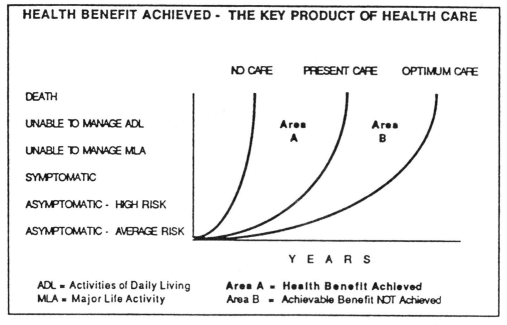

FIG 6–2.
Matrix figure illustrating patient outcome under three conditions: no care, present care, and optimum care. Health benefit is defined as a positive increment of any health care outcome measured on a value scale. (From Williamson JW, Moore DE, Sanazara PJ: *Eval Health Profess* 14:139–160, 1991. Used by permission.)

For example, can you take your treatment approaches for a specific therapeutic diagnosis category and graphically depict the changing health status of your patients? If you are unable to do this now, it is time to change your practice so this is possible in the future. The two curves may only be theoretical constructs based on your best judgment and information on (a) the natural history of the disease and (b) a given treatment's efficacy,[7] but it will allow you to begin to gauge and to critically assess the quality of your care and the remaining ABNA.

POSITION OF THE PROFESSION ON QUALITY ASSURANCE

The physical therapy profession through the American Physical Therapy Association (APTA) has for years taken a strong position on **quality assurance**. The evolution of quality assurance within the physical therapy profession and in external agencies has followed the move from small qa to LARGE QA. This effort began in 1972, when the APTA mandated chapter components to take responsibility in overseeing quality assurance activities of its members. The emphasis on *peer review* seen throughout these early years focused all quality assurance efforts on ensuring correct, timely documentation of our physical therapy processes and keeping adequate records to ensure minimum standards regarding the qualifications of staff were met (structure). An example of a model for peer review according to APTA Standards of Care is found in Appendix I–A. The APTA House of Delegates revised their policy statement on quality in 1985 and again in 1990. The present APTA policy statement, found in Appendix I–C does not specify the techniques that should be used or what part of the quality equation should be assessed. However, most experts in rehabilitation agree that any quality assurance or improvement efforts undertaken now should not only address the traditional *structure,* and *process* but also must include *outcome, content, and impact* as discussed in the previous section. In practice, however, many physical therapists only assess for structure and process components without having a true understanding of the outcome, content or impact of our care. It is important for us to continue to address small qa issues, but essential that we move on to the inclusion of LARGE QA techniques.

The need to ensure minimal competence and to comply with the quality assurance and credentialing standards of the external agencies (small qa) is sure to persist into the foreseeable future, even though these agencies are evolving and increasing their focus on accountability for LARGE QA activities.

Commonly recognized organizations that credential health care facilities and are known for monitoring standards include:

- Federal governmental agencies (Health Care Financing Administration, Medicare)
- State governmental agencies (DHHS, Medicaid)
- Professional associations (APTA)
- Independent accrediting agencies (Joint Commission on Accreditation of Healthcare Organizations [JCAHO],[9] Commission on Accreditation of Rehabilitation Facilities [CARF][10])

Let us examine how the changes in how these last two accrediting organizations have set standards relating to quality over the years.

JCAHO Agenda for Change

The JCAHO, formerly the Joint Commission on Accreditation of Hospitals (JCAH), began its efforts in the early 1970s with a traditional or "small qa" approach to standards for quality. The evolution of the standards by JCAHO is illustrated in Table 6–5.

The JCAHO began to acknowledge the shortcomings of its original approaches to quality care in the early 1980s. By 1987, it had introduced an Agenda for Change. This agenda called for all health care organizations accredited by the Commission to implement an "indicator monitoring system" accompanied by a quality improvement process. The JCAHO specified that the indicators chosen in any practice should relate to important specific aspects of care, safety issues, and customer satisfaction, all of which should be monitored on an ongoing basis. Today, the JCAHO regulations also spec-

TABLE 6–5.

Evolution of **JCAHO** Standards

small qa	Pre-1970s	Sets professional and accrediting agency standards
	1975	Promotes quality assurance audits (hospitals/JCAH)
	1980	Focuses on problem resolution (JCAH), and numerical requirements for audit eliminated
	1985	Fosters organization-wide program approach of ongoing quality assurance, stressing actions taken to evaluate effectiveness in improving patient care and problem resolution
	1990	Recognizes optimal continuous improvement in providing quality patient care
	1991	Stresses the value of services provided and outcomes achieved. Endorses Total Quality Management/Continuous Quality
LARGE QA		Improvement rather than early concepts of quality assurance

ify the number of indicators each service or discipline is required to monitor. Appendix IV–B shows JCAHO's recommended 10-Step Monitoring Process and provides general examples of indicators of care. This model begins the process of identifying and monitoring indicators over time and can be used in any setting to establish a quality monitoring system for specific indicators. The JCAHO Agenda for Change calls for pairing this routine monitoring effort with a system of quality improvement. The importance of this pairing cannot be overemphasized. The quality improvement process may be based in part of the JCAHO's current monitoring system but will require the organizations to examine the data gathered from the monitoring system and ask, "Is this the best we can do to improve the outcome of care?" Or, stated in the terminology of Williamson, "What is the ABNA (achievable benefits not achieved) for this type of patient or problem?"[7] The answers to these questions should force a reexamination and modification of the structure, process, or system of care to improve the outcome of care. Why should you as a therapist consider this type of quality improvement? First, for the good of the patient, and, second because the ever increasing managed care systems with which we all must deal value effective and efficient health care highly. Managed care systems are, by their actions, encouraging individual clinical centers to design TQM[11] programs in order to survive in a very competitive market.

Program Evaluation

The Commission on Accreditation of Rehabilitation Facilities (CARF) takes a different approach to assessing quality. The CARF approach, called Program Evaluation, is outcome based and is nationally recognized for its focus on the actual result of the rehabilitation program or service. The CARF defines Program Evaluation as a "systematic procedure for determining the results achieved by persons following the provision of services and determining the efficiency with which those results are obtained on a regular basis."[10] Program Evaluation provides individual therapists, department managers, or centers with a tool that can be used when making judgments about specific aspects of care relative to the total program or service. The process helps assess how a program is functioning, where additional resources are needed, and which issues need to be corrected. Program Evaluation is valuable for all practice settings, or at any level of care. It may be used with a single discipline or multiple services. It also can be used to assess consumer satisfaction and to look back at patient outcomes. Most practitioners hope that patients will return if they need similar services again and will share their enthusiasm for their treatment with people around them. The opportunity to improve the chances of this happening should be reason enough to make Program Evaluation an on-going quality assurance activity. The following is an example of the process of program evaluation.

1. Decide what is the critical problem or issue within your clinic that you want to study and improve.

   Earlier we mentioned a clinic that had 30% of its work-hardening patients fail to return to work. That clinic was the Work Hard PT Clinic. The fact that their rate of returning patients to work was only 70% was a problem for the clinic in its efforts to market its services. So this was the situation that Work Hard PT Clinic chose to study and improve through Program Evaluation.

2. Decide on an acceptable level or standard for your care.

   The manager of Work Hard, Don, on realizing the problem, re-viewed the literature to determine what were reasonable return to work rates. After poring through many studies Don determined that it would be acceptable if 5% of Work Hard's work-hardening patients did not return to work after treatment. Or, stated more positively, that 95% of their work-hardening patients would return to work in modified, transitional, or full duty within 8 weeks. His staff agreed.

3. Decide who you will need to talk to, to find out more background and information about the *possible causes of the problem*. This could include patients, family, other care givers, employers, and other involved persons or organizations.

   Don drafted some of the therapists in the clinic to assist in this effort. They decided to approach this situation as a team. They de-termined that they needed to talk to each individual therapist who worked in the work-hardening area, a sampling of work-hardening patients (they settled on 25), the front office personnel, the infor-mation systems specialist who may shed some light on any partic-ular trend related to those individuals who did not return to work or their therapy, the referring physicians, a sampling of employers whose injured employees were seen in the clinic, the vocational rehabilitation counselor who works with the clinic, a sampling of claims adjustors who worked with claims for the major employers, those occupational therapists involved in work hardening, and the psychologist who works with the program.

4. Decide what the key questions are that need to be asked in order to clarify the causes and identify possible solutions to the problem. It is important when asking questions to only inquire about things you don't know. Your purpose is to probe to the true cause (structure, process, content).

Don determined his questions by putting the name of each person he needed to talk to on a sheet of paper and listing all the things that the individual could answer that Don did not know about the care. His list for the information specialist began
- Did the patients who did not return to work have anything in common, such as a similar therapist, a similar referral source, a similar employer, a similar diagnosis, a similar job or a similar attorney?
- How were these factors different than the total patient population in work hardening?
- Was there a significant variation in the timeliness of their referral after the initial date of injury compared with the patients in work hardening who had returned to work?
- Was there a significant variation in the course of treatment for those patients who did not return to work compared to those who did as seen from billing records?

5. Decide what your actions plan will be based on the results of your study.

After over a month and a half of extensive interviewing, probing, and researching, Don and his cadre of helpers from the department determined that two major factors were influencing the return to work status of their patients. The first was a delay in referral to work hardening. The second was a variation in technique they discovered: two therapists had not attended any formal course work in work hardening, and their patients consistently did not make the same type of objective progress as did the patients of therapists with this training. The team then developed a detailed course of action for each of these problems. In this action plan, they designated the action, the party responsible for initiating action, the timeline for completion of action, and the person who would monitor the activity for completion. Using Program Evaluation, they believed they had resolved the problem.

One of the strong features in Program Evaluation is that it is possible to redo the study in the future if the questions posed are such that they repeatedly need current answers. In the case example, Don did decide to reexamine the return to work rate for all therapists in 7 months to see if the actions they had put in place had effected any change and indeed resolved the problem. In previous sections of this chapter, definitions for quality care were outlined and current ways of assessing quality care both within the profession and by external agencies were discussed.

The following section deals with implementing, modifying, or strengthening your current method of ensuring and improving quality care.

SELF ASSESSMENT

We begin with a quality assurance self assessment (Fig 6–3). As you can see from this flow sheet diagram, resolution of the problems that affect the quality of the care within your clinic or department is a prime reason for

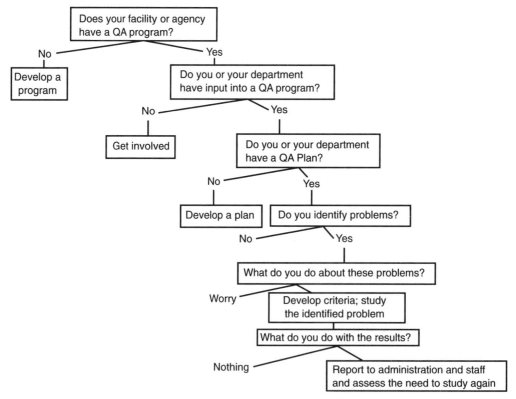

FIG 6–3.
Decision tree to be used by each practice to determine extent of quality assurance/improvement activities.

quality management efforts. Another key reason presents itself when all of the major problems or crises are resolved and the practice must maintain or improve its current "quality care" performance.

Step 1: Identify Problems

The first step in beginning quality management in your practice setting is to identify the problems or situations within your clinic that affect the quality of your care. Despite traditional quality assurance word choice, we will call all these problems opportunities. One thing that should be apparent by now is that each of the parties that have a stake in the care of the patient has a different opinion regarding what constitutes quality care. We believe it is critical that each of these stakeholder's opinions related to quality care and their perceptions about your clinic *must* be taken into consideration when you go about identifying the problem or situation to be addressed in your QM efforts. Some of the major stakeholders we identified earlier in this chapter are the patient, the provider, the employer/payer, and utilization review firms. One previously unmentioned is the referral source.

The Patient (Consumer)

Earlier in the chapter, we discussed patient's perceptions (in general) related to quality care. We believe these can be distilled down to *two fundamental characteristics* that must exist if the patient (the consumer) is to believe quality care has occurred:

1. The care has generally improved the health status of the patient in ways the patient considers important
2. The care has generated patient satisfaction or has met or exceeded patient expectations for the treatment

How do you know if your patients consider these aspects important? Ask them! The best way to determine the critical determinants of quality in your patient population is to read the scientifically based research, which we have attempted to share with you, and to verify such information within your practice environment. How do you ask? You could do a survey, ask pertinent questions of a small but representative sampling of your patients, or conduct a formal or informal focus group of patients. One physician has, by his own report, markedly improved his practice and the alliance of his patients by calling together a group of his patients' parents (he is a pediatrician) semiannually or annually and having an informal focus group to discuss the areas of his practice that are most difficult for his patients (and parents) and cooperatively talk about solutions that will remedy or at least mitigate the situations.[12]

For the sake of discussion, we will assume that your patients' responses agree with the research presented earlier in this chapter. If this is the case, how then do you determine if the majority of your patients believe these two characteristics of quality exist in your practice? A number of possibilities exist. Perhaps the easiest way is through the use of intake and discharge questionnaires (Figs 6–4 and 6–5). Figure 6–3 is a modification of a traditional intake questionnaire to include patient rating of their perceived abilities to complete functional tasks. Of those they believe they are unable to perform at the time of intake, the tool requests they rate the level of that task's importance. The form uses segments from Allen's scale discussed in Chapter 4. If this is completed upon intake, the therapist will be able to utilize the information readily when setting, with the patient, the functional goals for the course of treatment. It will also serve to compare and contrast the patient's expectations of therapy with the expectations of the therapist. Entering therapy with a realistic expectation for treatment should have many positive effects. The results of this functional rating section of the intake questionaire will then be compared to the results from the functional segment of the Patient Satisfaction Questionnaire and correlated to the general patient satisfaction score. This survey should not only be handed to patients at their last visit with a stamped return envelope but it should be sent to all patients who have failed to return to therapy for three consecutive treatments or 3 weeks. The results from these two tools should provide your clinic with information on whether your patients are generally satisfied with care and if they feel that they have improved their health or functional status as a result of therapy. If they are less than satisfied or they do not overwhelmingly perceive that they have improved their health status, you have identified a problem, opportunity, or situation that should be addressed within your quality management efforts. Additional areas that would be beneficial to include within these tools are measurements of patient pain, as reported along a visual analog scale or other objective measure; general health status and general psychological health (a tool we would recommend for this is Interstudy's "SF-36" (Short Form with 36 questions); and TyPE instruments (Technology of Patient Experience) administered prior to treatment and after treatment.[13]

Providers

The professional (provider) in general considers quality care as care that generates therapist or staff satisfaction; care that is provided by the same therapist or practitioner; or care that meets the standard of care in their com-

PATIENT INTAKE FORM

Patient Name _____

Address _____

Phone   Home (___)_____ Work (___)_____

What problems brought you to Physical Therapy?_____
_____

What were you able to do before that you can't do now?_____
_____

For each of the following activities, please place a check in the appropriate box. If **No/Not Well** has been checked, please indicate how important it is to perform better on this activity as a result of therapy.

R a t i n g s: 1- Not at all important
2 - Somewhat important
3 - Moderately important
4 - Very important
5 - Extremely important

Can Perform

Activity/Functional Skills	YES	NO/Not Well	Rating	Activity/Function	YES	NO/Not Well	Rating
Sitting				Using the Stairs			
Standing for up to ____ mins/hr				Dressing			
Rolling				Grooming			
Transfer to/from bath				Can prepare and serve food			
Bathing				Using phone			
Transfer to/from car				Shopping			
Driving				Managing children			
Walking at home				Lifting			
Walking in neighborhood				Carrying			
Walking in community				Reaching			
Accessing buildings				Stooping/Squatting			

Have you been treated or are you currently being treated by a physician or other health care practitioner for any medical or physical problems? _____ If so, what are they?_____
_____

What medications are you taking, if any?_____
_____

What allergies do you have, if any?_____
_____

Do you have any new complaints or problems? _____
_____
_____

Signature _____   Date _____

FIG 6–4.
Patient intake questionnaire that incorporates a modified version of Allen's scale to assess patient's perception of their function. This may be used later for quality assessment of care received. (Courtesy of Elizabeth Gaynor, P.T., Hartsdale, N.Y.)

┌─────────────────────────────┐
│ **PATIENT SATISFACTION SURVEY** │
└─────────────────────────────┘

Tell us what you think so we can serve you better!

Consider the following statements and circle the face on the scale that best represents the way you feel toward each statement.

Appointments were scheduled for me quickly.

I rarely had to wait more than 5 minutes for treatment.

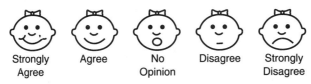

The therapist understood my goals and we developed short-term goals and overall goals together.

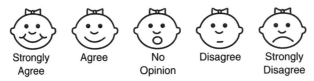

The therapist spent enough time with me and answered my questions fully and in terms that I could understand.

The clinic's policies were explained to me in terms that I understood.

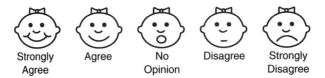

FIG 6–5.
Simplified patient discharge questionnaire that assesses patient satisfaction and perception of functional abilities. This can be used in conjunction with the patient intake questionnaire (see Fig 6–3). (Courtesy of First Physical Therapy, Billings, Mont., and Baton Rouge Physical Therapy, Baton Rouge, La.)

The business office was pleasant and helpful to me.

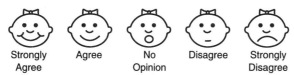

| Strongly Agree | Agree | No Opinion | Disagree | Strongly Disagree |

My account statements from the clinic were understandable and itemized correctly.

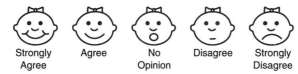

| Strongly Agree | Agree | No Opinion | Disagree | Strongly Disagree |

The treatment I received at the clinic was effective in meeting my goals.

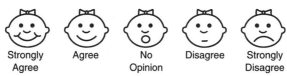

| Strongly Agree | Agree | No Opinion | Disagree | Strongly Disagree |

For each of the following activities, please place a check in the appropriate box. If **No/Not Well** has been checked, please indicate how much better you can perform this activity as a result of therapy.

R a t i n g s:
1 - Not at all improved
2 - Somewhat improved
3 - Moderately improved
4 - Very improved
5 - Extremely improved

Can Perform **Activity/Functional** Skills	YES	NO/Not Well	Rating	Activity/Function	YES	NO/Not Well	Rating
Sitting				Using the Stairs			
Standing for up to ____ min/hr				Dressing			
Rolling				Grooming			
Transfer to/from bath				Can prepare and serve food			
Bathing				Using phone			
Transfer to/from car				Shopping			
Driving				Managing children			
Walking at home				Lifting			
Walking in neighborhood				Carrying			
Walking in community				Reaching			
Accessing buildings				Stooping/Squatting			

My therapist was: _____

THANK YOU FOR COMPLETING THIS QUESTIONNAIRE AND FOR LETTING US BE OF SERVICE TO YOU...

Pauline Practitioner, P.T.
President

FIG 6-5 (cont.).

munity, region, or nation. What do the therapists in your practice believe equates to quality care? If you do not know the answer to this, we have included a questionnaire titled Survey on Quality in Physical Therapy in Appendix IV–A, which you can use to survey their feelings and perceptions. The results of this simple survey may point out one problem, opportunity, or situation that is in need of improvement if your practice is to move toward the future well-positioned for success.

Payer/Employer/Adjuster

Consistently, payers, and employers have stated that the most important quality care issues in their viewpoint are that

- Care generates patient/employee satisfaction
- Care leads to quantifiable functional improvement within the limits of reimbursement, lowers the total work days lost due to an injury or illness, or makes the maximum possible contribution to the reduction of lost productivity (that is, the care received is effective and cost-efficient)
- Care is appropriately and completely documented

These factors appear in Tables 6–1 and Figure 6–1 as well as in all of the literature that discusses business and health issues. Who are the major employers and payers in your practice? How many of their group health and Workers' Compensation patients have you seen in the past 2 years? Is that number up or down from the preceding 2 years? Do you ever communicate with them, ask their opinion on your services, question the effectiveness of your care? This can be done in a survey mode similar to that discussed for patients and providers, or you can develop an Industrial Advisory Council of key representatives from employers. These councils can provide input on what your town's employers believe to be the critical factors for quality health care, provide input on your performance as a clinic in delivering these quality elements, and perhaps even assist you in developing an action plan to help you meet their quality demands. From that one council (through perhaps several meetings) you will not only have built a long-term relationship with a key stakeholder in your patient's care but you will have also identified critical quality management issues and probably a number of possible solutions as well.

Referral Source

It is difficult to determine which of the key elements for quality care affect the referral source. We postulate that these individuals perceive quality care to exist when the care provided

- Leads to improved clinical outcome or generally improved the health status of the patient
- Leads to patient satisfaction

However, other factors may influence their perceptions, such as the frequency of reports, the rate of return to their clinic of the patients they refer to your clinic, your availability, and so forth. The only way to know where you stand with this critical stakeholder in the care of your patients is to ask. Have an outside agency ask for you. Have a friend act as an outside agency and mail the results of an inquiry back to you. It is critical to quality improvement and quality management that you establish baseline data and search hard to identify possible problems or opportunities for improvement and then strive to improve them.

The last method we will discuss for identifying any possible quality management or quality improvement problems within your clinic is to examine your practices routinely through a peer review format to see if the treatments provided for each patient or class of patients are those that are

- *Efficacious* according to the literature (in other words, the treatment techniques you are using should have been demonstrated in research to have been effective)
- *Appropriate* for the patient's condition
- *Executed* with the best technique and procedures possible.

Step 2: Selecting and Defining the Highest Priority Problem(s)/ Opportunities for Improvement

After the baseline information from each of the stakeholders has been gathered, we suggest that a "quality circle" be formed to look at, analyze, and work to solve work-related quality of service and quality of work life issues. The usual size for a quality circle is six to eight people. The members meet voluntarily with a group leader and facilitator. This group reviews the perceptions on the practice's quality of care obtained from each stakeholder. They would then set acceptable goals or levels of performance for each area. These goals should be stated objectively and clearly so it will be apparent to all when the goals are met. Let us look at two examples. A clinic whose patient satisfaction goal stated simply, "The monthly results from a patient survey will be positive," would have difficulty deciding when this goal is obtained. Will they have achieved their goal when 100% of the questions were answered with the best possible smiley face, or when 51% of the questionnaires have 51% of the questions answered with no unhappy faces? This goal is unclear, and therapists will not likely be motivated to achieve it. The clinic down the road, on the other hand, has stated their patient satisfaction goal statement as, Each therapist should have a patient satisfaction average score rating greater than 4 (the fourth smiley face from the right) and a rate of returns of survey from patients of over 50%. If any survey returned averages 5, the therapist responsible will receive two bonus points. For each 10 bonus points the therapist receives a half-day off with pay.

After objective goals are set, the quality group should prioritize the problems/opportunities and the goals. They may ask questions such as: How important is this problem/goal? How much control over the goal does the circle have? How can success be measured?[3] Within this brainstorming discussion, the circle should remember the short-term and long-term goals of the practice and its basic organization philosophy.

Step 3: Analyze Key Problem(s)/Opportunity for Improvement

With a prioritized list of opportunities and goals in hand, the quality circle should begin to completely analyse the most critical problem or problems. It is critical in this stage to get input from any person who may have an insight into the problem area. When discussing program evaluation earlier in this chapter, we listed some of the people that Don, the manager of the Work Hard Clinic, would need to talk to about one problem. This list was extensive. The quality circle cannot attempt to analyze and determine the true causes of the problems isolated from the people who are actively involved in the problem area or without looking at the entire step-by-step process that leads to the situation. A number of different techniques exist to analyze problems. One such technique can be found in the Model for Peer Review/APTA Standards (Appendix IV–C).

Step 4: Develop Solutions

At this step, members of the quality circle, together with key personnel who are involved in the process, should begin to brainstorm solutions to the problems identified. All solutions should be written and then reviewed in search of the best one or two solutions. When they are finalized, each solution should have a time line associated with it as well as a person designated to be responsible for implementing the solution. We have found it useful to also include a party responsible for monitoring the activity.

Step 5: Implement and Monitor

Once the plan is developed, the time has come to implement the plan. If the quality circle does not have this authority, they must present their findings, conclusions, and suggested actions with a rationale for implementation to those who do have authority. Once the implementation has occurred, it is important to monitor the effectiveness of the solutions at routine intervals. For example: Assume your problem was a poor referral source satisfaction with the outcomes they perceived as a result of your care. Your investigation and analysis led you to determine that the physicians did not understand the reports you were sending or that your reports were frequently not sent to them on a timely basis. The solution developed by the quality team in your practice was a modified reporting format that was to be completed by the tenth of each month by each therapist for each patient and forwarded immediately to the referral source. Three months after the clinic had implemented this solution, a repeat survey of the physicians revealed that their opinions had not changed. Although they liked the new report format and that you were sending timely reports, the reports were still not entered into the physicians' charts. What to do? Reexamine the problem, this time with the focus on finding a different way to assure the information contained within the report found its way to the physicians for review when the patients visit their physicians. You might try motivating the physicians' office staffs to immediately file your reports in the appropriate patients chart, faxing the report (faxes are often perceived to be more of a critical nature than U.S. mail), presenting the information to the physician yourself at rounds, providing a copy to the patient to take with them for their visit, or calling the results to the doctor. But the monitoring of the effectiveness of the solution must continue until you are assured that the problem has really been resolved.

In summary the six steps are as follows:

1. Identify problems
2. Select and define the highest priority problems
3. Analyze the problem
4. Create a solution
5. Implement the solutions
6. Monitor.[3] A format we have used in reports using this approach to quality management, starting with step two in the process, is shown in Table 6–6.

We have presented you with a wide array of definitions on quality and a method for assessing quality. Developing a quality assurance–quality man-

TABLE 6–6.

FORMAT TO MONITORING QUALITY MANAGEMENT EFFORTS

Problem/Opportunity	Cause	Solution	Responsible Party	Timeline	Monitoring Party
Physician's poor perception of outcome	Content and timeliness of reports	Modify reports Reports due by the 10th of month	Department Manager, with input from team	4/1/93	Quality Committee

agement plan provides you with a process through which there can be systematic and objective monitoring and evaluation of the appropriateness of care provided. Defining what constitutes quality for the organization is a beginning. The commitment for quality must come from the top in the conceptual chain-of-command framework. It is our hope that you will see that the outcome of your care is a critical and that by maintaining quality management activities you will position your practice for the future. By having your own plan you can address critical issues unique to your center, such as

- Right treatment at the right time by the right person
- Communication (written/verbal) clear, and as needed by constituent
- Risk-free services and environment
- Competitive with other providers
- All staff involved in the plan to provide total and continuous quality care
- Meet professional and community or organization standards
- Best patient care outcomes, at a competitive cost when care is medically necessary
- Identify important aspects of care for your clinical center, such as
  Referrals
  Initial evaluation
  Performance of procedures
  Plan of care
  Reevaluation/progression of patient in terms of outcome

REFERENCES

1. *Websters' Ninth New Collegiate Dictionary*, 1984, s.v. "quality."
2. Berwick DM: Health services research and quality of care assignments for the 1990's, *Med Care* 27:763–771, 1989.

3. *Quality Assurance: An APTA Practice Management Publication.* Alexandria, Va, 1990, American Physical Therapy Association.

4. Joint Commission. Quality Review Bulletin, Journal of Quality Improvement. Joint Commission on Accreditation of Health Organizations, Chicago, Illinois. Vol 18, No 1. January 1992, pg 2.

5. Joint Commission on Accreditation of Healthcare Organizations: Development of guidelines; QRB—quality review bulletin, *J Quality Improvement* 12:19, 1991.

6. Mooney G: *Economics, The Road to Better Physiotherapy;* London, WCPT, July 1991, pp 1567–1572.

7. Williamson JW, Moore DE, Sanazara PJ: Moving from "small qa" to "large QA": an outcomes framework for improving quality management. *Eval Health Profess* 14:139–160, 1991.

8. de Gyndt W: Five approaches for assessing the quality of care. *Hosp Admin* 159;21–42, 1970.

9. *The Joint Commission 1991 Accreditation Manual for Hospitals,* Chicago, 1990, Joint Commission on Accreditation of Healthcare Organizations.

10. *Standards Manual for Organizations Serving People with Disabilities,* Tucson, Arizona, 1989, Commission on Accreditation of Rehabilitation Facilities.

11. Walton M: *The Deming management method.* New York, 1986, Perigee Book, Putnam Publishing.

12. Attwood CR: Give these little extras and watch your practice grow. *Med Economics* March 2, 1992.

13. Interstudy: Outcomes Management System (OMS), Excelsior, Minn, 1991.

TEST YOUR KNOWLEDGE

1. Quality in health care is difficult to define. List four entities that may have a stake in the definition, then compare and contrast their differing definitions.
2. A physician from the Harvard Community Health Plan has put forth four "pillars" of quality. List and discuss each of these.
3. Discuss guideline or algorithm development and its role in quality management.
4. List and discuss five critical functional areas that should be used when measuring quality.
5. Compare quality assurance and quality improvement.
6. Identify the ABNA concept in health care quality improvement as discussed by Williamson et al. Discuss this concept and its possible effect on physical therapy.
7. Discuss the Joint Commission on Accreditation of Healthcare Organization 10-Step model.
8. Outline the five-step process for quality improvement in health care and give an example of its use. Try to incorporate your answer to question 1 in this response.

TEST YOUR KNOWLEDGE ANSWER SHEET

1. a. Professionals perceive quality when they:
    (1) Can practice current state of the profession.
    (2) Have autonomy.
    (3) Can provide the patient with optimal care.
    b. Consumers perceive quality when practitioners:
    (1) Quickly recognize consumers perceived needs.
    (2) Are courteous and communicate concern.
    c. Consumers perceive quality when consumers:
    (1) Get better with care provided.
    (2) Are able to function and return to vocation/avocation.
    d. Third-party payers perceive quality when there is:
    (1) Efficient, effective use of funds.
    (2) Client satisfaction.
    (3) Clients return to work/functional level.

Another way to summarize each stakeholder's perception of quality is as follows:

1. *Professionals (providers)* generally consider quality care that which generates therapist or staff satisfaction, is provided by the same therapist or practitioner, or meets the standard of care in the community/region/nation.
2. *Patient:* Two fundamental characteristics must exist if the patient (consumer) is to believe quality care has been received:
   a. The care has generally improved health status in ways the patient considers important.
   b. The care generated patient satisfaction or met or exceeded patient expectations for the treatment.
3. *Payers, employers, adjusters* consistently state that the most important criteria of quality care are:
   a. The care generated patient or employee satisfaction.
   b. The care leads to quantifiable functional improvement within the limits of reimbursement, lowers the total work days lost due to an injury or illness, or makes the maximum possible contribution to the reduction of lost productivity (i.e., the care is effective and cost-efficient).
4. *Referral source:* The referral source is usually difficult to assess regarding key elements of quality care. We postulate that these persons perceive quality care to exist when the care provided:
   a. Leads to improved clinical outcome or generally improves the health status of the patient.

b. Leads to patient satisfaction.
5. Donald Berwick of the Harvard Community Health Plan has proposed four pillars of quality and quality research:
    a. *Efficacy* of care practices, or knowing what works.
    b. *Appropriateness* of decisions, or using what works.
    c. *Execution* of care, or doing well what works.
    d. *Purpose* of care, or clarifying the values that tell us what we wish to do.
6. A great deal of attention is currently being focused on improving the decision-making process in patient care. Improved decision-making studies generally favor highly structured methods and endorse explicit estimation over implicit judgment. Because of this, many have begun to develop community standards, guidelines, or algorithms of care. These community standards and algorithms and guidelines are, in Berwick's opinion, "a convenient way to convey existing scientific data into action. When scientific data are lacking, they can be conscientious best guesses, (and therefore) are better than the random variation" of practice.[2] Algorithms and/or guidelines simply specify appropriate care based on research, expert judgment, and practice environment. They allow us to provide better health care by facilitating scientific review. Because guidelines or algorithms usually are developed to reduce variation from practice to practice; to reduce uncertainty about quality, efficacy, and effectiveness; and to reformat existing information that could improve clinical decision making but is not now in an easily usable format, they are useful in quality management efforts.
7. The five areas that should be included in quality management efforts are:
    a. Structure: measurement of qualifications of staff, physical structure, licensure, professional credentials.
    b. Process: measurement of what the health care practitioner does.
    c. Outcome: Measurement of patient outcome.
    d. Content: measurement of appropriateness of care (utilization).
    e. Impact: measurement of effect of care on society.
8. Quality assurance and quality improvement may be compared as follows:

Small qa (Quality Assurance)	Large qa (Quality Improvement)
Program	Process
Coordinator/Director, Committee driven	Management driven
No historical value for customer input	Consumer driven
Assign responsibility for monitoring	Organize knowledgeable team
Delineate scope of care and identify most important aspects of care	Find a process improvement opportunity

Systematic monitoring based on indicators	Clarify current knowledge of process
Establish thresholds; focus on special causes	Strive for (continuous improvement), reduce variation
Monitor care by collecting and organizing date indicator	Uncover root causes of variation
Evaluate care when thresholds indicates that one should improve care or identify problem	Start improvement cycle

9. ABNA is the acronym for Achievable Benefits Not Achieved. Williamson et al. propose that this is the difference between the progression of the disability under optimal conditions of care and the progression of the disability with care currently received. They state that this should be the major focus of LARGE QA activities. For each treatment intervention undertaken, this theory proposes that a therapist look at the short-term and long-term differences between these two factors as well as the difference between the progression of the disability if no care was provided and under optimal and current care. By taking this approach, a provider should look at the effectiveness of the treatment intervention (by conducting a comparison of current care and no intervention) and at the opportunity for quality improvement (by comparing progression with current care and with optimal care). Effectiveness and quality improvement are two important factors in any quality management system.

10. The JCAHO 10-Step monitoring process is a problem-solving model that can be used in any setting to establish a quality monitoring process. It focuses on the monitoring of care through the use of indicators. Indicators relate to specific aspects of care, safety issues, and customer satisfaction. Within this system each indicator must have a threshold for performance. Thresholds are different from goals in that goals are what you strive for and thresholds are realistically what occurs. The 10-step process is as follows:
   a. Assign responsibility.
   b. Delineate scope of service.
   c. Identify important aspects of care.
   d. Identify indicators.
   e. Set thresholds for evaluation.
   f. Collect and organize data.
   g. Evaluate care.
   h. Take action, solve problems.
   i. Assess actions, document improvement.
   j. Communicate information to quality assurance/quality improvement program.

11. One quality improvement process is the use of the five-step process:
   a. Identify problems.
   b. Select and define the highest priority problems.

c. Analyze the problem(s).
d. Create a solution(s).
e. Implement the solutions and monitor.

For example: A clinic (Work Hard) identifies through their preliminary marketing efforts for their functional capacity evaluations that the local employers have minimal knowledge about their clinic. In the rare instance, they do indicate they know something about the clinic, they state they heard that the clinic is a "mill." For a clinic that is trying to gather more business referrals this is a problem. Don, the clinic's administrator, decides to clarify this problem first. He invites 15 of the local employers to a luncheon meeting at the clinic to talk about their needs and expectations. During the meeting he also further explores these employers' perceptions of Work Hard. What Don discovers is that the employers' perceptions about the quality of care at Work Hard are based on reports from their claims examiners. After the meeting, Don sits down with his staff to discuss this problem. By the end of the discussion they have defined the problem specifically and created a plan to gather information to analyze the problem. This plan required that a meeting similar to the employer meeting take place with the examiners, and if this were impossible, a representative from the clinic would meet with a representative sampling of examiners. More than 30 days of effort went into gathering information for analysis. Then the staff and Don sat down to brainstorm. On discussing the situation, it became clear that the examiners did not feel the information that Work Hard was providing assisted them in completing their tasks. A solution was then apparent: reformat their reporting to meet the examiners' needs. The methodology to do this was developed, then implemented. In addition, the Work Hard staff decided to monitor the examiners' feelings about their new reporting for a further 90 days to determine if their solution was effective.

GLOSSARY

Activity restriction   Defines a functional limitation or disability in terms of specific tasks or activities that can be measured or monitored.

ABNA   (Achievable benefits not achieved). Terminology proposed by Williamson et al.[8] to designate the difference between progression of a disability under optimal conditions of care and progression of the disability with care currently received. These authors state that ABNA should be the major focus of LARGE QA activities.

Americans With Disabilities Act (ADA)   This Act, signed into law on July 26, 1990, provides comprehensive civil rights protection to individuals with disabilities in the areas of employment, public accommodations, state and local government services, and telecommunications. Of specific interest to physical therapists are the definitions and nomenclature regarding disability.

Algorithms of care   These algorithms, often seen as flow charts or decision trees (see Chapter 2), provide a convenient way to convey existing scientific data into action, and are seen as standards for appropriate care based on research, expert opinion, and varying practice environments.

Beneficiary   Term used to describe the patient in the claims review process.

Commission on Accreditation of Rehabilitation Facilities (CARF)   Accreditation agency for rehabilitation facilities, either within a hospital setting or a free-standing facility.

Community standard   Community-specific standards for appropriate care based on research, expert opinion, and varying practice environments.

Comprehensive Outpatient Rehabilitation Facility (CORF)   Facility must meet standards for certification as set forth by the Commission on Accreditation of Rehabilitation Facilities.

Capitation   Flat fee paid regardless of number of services provided.

Carrier   Insurance company that writes coverage. A carrier may also review Medicare claims submitted by a client, physician, or other health care provider to determine if a claim is reasonable and necessary based on Medicare law.

Competition   Market strategy in which providers of care compete for volume of referrals through competitive pricing with other providers.

Composite activities   Number of coordinated task elements and tasks that meet a personal or social need (e.g., driving, materials handling, shopping, personal hygiene).

Certificate of need (CON)   Part of the regulatory process imposed in the 1970s to control expansion of facilities and technology.

Concurrent review   Traditionally used to define a review that occurs at the same time as medical care is being provided. This type of review is frequently viewed as a way to evaluate length of stay, appropriateness of services, and discharge planning for patients in acute care facilities. It may also be applied to review of care in other patient care settings.

Content   Measurement of the appropriateness of care (utilization).

Control   That era of health care evolution focused on constraining health care costs through regulation.

Co-payment   Type of cost sharing in which a fixed amount is paid by the insured for each service (e.g., $5 for an office visit).

Corrected incentives   Term created during the period when attempts were made to reorganize the health care delivery system to promote efficiency. System designs were developed to create health maintenance organizations and preferred provider organizations.

Coordinated care   Organized process that includes all services provided to a patient from hospital admission to final discharge either to a less costly alternative center or to the home environment. It is the essence of discharge planning to assure that the patient receives continued follow-up in planning for his or her health needs. Important in Managed Care.

Deductible(s)   Form of cost sharing in which the patient must pay for services out-of-pocket before payment is made by the insurer.

Department of Health and Human Services (DHHS)   Federal agency that oversees Medicaid programs (Title XIX of the Social Security Act). Medicaid is jointly funded by state and federal governments and is administered at the state level. It provides health care benefits for elderly, disabled, and poor. Each state may choose to pay more than the federally mandated minimum.

Design defects   Specific design in a delivery system that is interfering with cost containment, such as the retrospective payment design.

Diagnosis Related Groups (DRGs)   Classification system used by Medicare for determination of hospital charges on the basis of patient diagnosis, complicating or co-morbid conditions, need for surgery, age, sex, and discharge status. A fixed amount is paid for each discharged patient depending on the assigned DRG.

Disability   Any restriction (resulting from impairment) of ability to perform an activity in the manner or within the range considered normal. Compare Functional disability; Functional limitation; Impairment.

Discounted rates   Provider agrees to provide a service at a percentage of the usual and customary costs.

Discrete measurements   Specific, quantifiable measurements of impairment, not function, that result from a traditionally reported evaluation (e.g., range of motion measurements, manual muscle test scores).

Dysfunction   Within the Functional Outcome Report (FOR) model, the direct effect of an impairment on an element of a task.

Economic indicators   Status of national financial resources that influence health care policy (e.g., inflation, budget deficit).

Economics   Use of resources so as to ensure that society gets the best possible return in terms of human welfare from available resources.

Edits   Listing of diagnoses in the Medicare guidelines that prescribes a set number of visits per illness and duration of treatment in terms of months.

Efficiency   Performing at a maximum level of productivity with minimal expenditure of resources.

Elements of tasks   In the physical sense, simple movements without sequence or purpose (e.g., reaching, stepping, sit to stance).

Explicit estimation   Decision-making process so plain and distinct that there is no need for inference and no difficulty in understanding it.

Findings   Result of valuative techniques.

Flagged   Medical charts or records that do *not* meet requirements for immediate payment or that fall within previously specified "exception" guidelines are flagged for further review. These initial requirements for payment and exception guidelines are often developed by and specific to each carrier or third-party payer.

Functional outcome   As defined by Blue Cross of California, patient status after therapy must meet three criteria: meaningful outcome, utilitarian outcome, and sustained outcome. *Meaningful outcome* is one in which the activity level achieved by the patient as a result of physical therapy is that level necessary for the patient to function most effectively at home or at work. *Practical outcome* represents the most economical and efficient method by which to perform the desired activity. *Sustained outcome* demonstrates that the activity level achieved is maintained outside the clinical environment and over a period of time.

Functional disability   Restriction or inability to perform normal activities of daily living.

Functional limitation   Loss of function best described, not by impairment, but in terms of activity restrictions or altered task performance.

Gatekeeper/gatekeeping   Control mechanism for utilization of health care services by means of physician review in order to control costs.

Gross National Product (GNP)   Sum of the dollar value of all goods and services produced in a country in 1 year. GNP is used as a measure of the state of the economy and the relative wealth of the society.

Guidelines   Standards for appropriate care based on research, expert opinion, and varying practice environments.

Handicap   As defined by the World Health Organization, a handicap is a disadvantage resulting from an impairment or disability, that limits or prevents fulfillment of a role that is normal, depending on age, sex, and social and cultural factors. Also, a classification of circumstances in which disabled people are likely to find themselves. Handicap describes the social and economic roles of impaired or disabled persons that place them at a disadvantage when compared with other persons. These disadvantages are a result of the interaction of the person with specific environments and cultures. Examples of handicaps that are relevant to this book include being bedridden or confined to home, inability to use public transportation, not working, underemployment, and social isolation.

Health Care Finance Administration (HCFA)   Government agency that oversees Medicare programs (Title XVIII of Social Security Act). Medicare is a federally funded program intended to cover certain health care costs for persons 65 years of age and older or designated disabled people younger than 65 years.

Health Maintenance Organization (HMO)   Insurance program in which the enrollee pays a fixed fee and in return receives a specific set of health care benefits.

Health Systems Agency (HSA)   Regulatory control implemented by Congress to enhance health planning at the local level and to control costs through systematic coordinated planning nationwide.

Household share   That share of the cost of paying for health care that is the responsibility of the individual for self and family. May be insurance premiums or out-of-pocket expenses.

IDC-9 **codes**   International classification of diseases developed by the World Health Organization. These codes are used as a tool for indexing medical records, medical care review, and ambulatory and other medical care programs. The codes classify diagnoses, which are used for reporting diagnoses and disease in all U.S. Public Health Service and Health Care Finance Administration programs. These codes, or similar codes such as CPT codes, are used by carriers to edit or screen claims for reimbursement of services. They must appear on claims submitted as a part of the determination of reasonable and necessary care based on the diagnostic classification.

Impact   Measurement of effect on society.

Impairment   As defined by the World Health Organization, any loss or abnormality of psychologic, physiologic, or anatomic structure or function. Impairments are disturbances at the level of an organ (e.g., defects in or loss of limb, organ, or other body structure) as well as defects or loss of mental function.

Implicit judgment   Judgment required when the link between two variables (e.g., being present in a class; a complete understanding of the subject matter presented) is not revealed, expressed, or developed.

Independent Physicians Associations (IPAs)   Organization composed of physicians who have collectively organized for the purpose of contracting with prepaid health plans (HMOs, PPOs) and other third-party payers.

Indicators   Identified occurrences that warrant investigation, an outlier compared with peers, or a sentinel event.

Intermediary   Insurance entity that reviews Medicare claims submitted by hospitals or other providers and determines whether a claim is reasonable and necessary based on Medicare law.

Linear progression   Easily followed logical progression from identified problem to proposed treatment.

Managed care   Any form of health plan that uses concepts of selective contracting to channel patients to a limited number of providers and that requires utilization review as a means to control unnecessary use of health care services. Also called Coordinated Care.

Market dynamics   General term for activities that influence the balance of resources and demand.

Meaningful outcome   Outcome that allows the patient to function most effectively at home or at work.

Medicaid   Federal- and state-funded entitlement program to subsidize health care for the indigent and poor.

Medical-impairment model   Disease-oriented approach to reducing or eliminating the manifestations of a disease or injury process. This model suggests that impairments are not only the result of disease but also its final expression.

Medicare   Federally funded supplemental health care coverage for persons 65 years or older and for the disabled. Recipients of Medicare must be eligible for Social Security or be the spouse of someone who is.

Medicare Part A   Insurance that covers inpatient hospital care, inpatient skilled nursing care, home health care, and hospice care.

Medicare Part B   Insurance coverage for physician services, outpatient hospital services, durable medical equipment, and other services and supplies not covered by Medicare Part A. Insured must pay a monthly premium to receive coverage.

Menu options   Employees may select from a menu of health care benefit plans that offer a variety of services and decide what coverage best meets individual and family needs based on the cost of premiums.

Mitigation Any attempt to decrease or reduce the extent of financial loss during provision of services.

Movement dysfunction Direct effect or effects of an impairment on a movement element of a task. A movement dysfunction could be the basis for the person's activity restriction.

Negligence Legally actionable careless treatment resulting in injury to a patient. Four elements must exist to some degree for negligence to be proved. The extent to which all four elements can be proved determines the extent of malpractice if one is called to court or sued. The four elements are (1) the physical therapist owed the patient a duty of care, (2) the physical therapist breached that duty of care, (3) the patient was injured, and (4) the injury was a result of the physical therapist's breach of duty of care.

Negotiated fees Fees decided on by payers and providers for the delivery of health care services. Usually these fees are lower than usual and customary fees.

Other health care services Category of personal health care services that includes dental, drug, physical therapy, occupational therapy, and other non–primary care services.

Outcome Status of the patient after care has been provided; end result of care. Outcomes should be written as time-specific, measurable, and in functional terms.

Outcome assessment Process of evaluation based on the predicted functional outcome of services provided.

Outcome management Concept introduced by Paul M. Ellwood for gathering and analyzing data that show the results of medical processes and performances, then using that data to manage the provision of health care. Most experts believe that consistent use of outcome management will change the incentives in the health care system to reward efficiency and effectiveness in delivery of services.

Payment subsidies Financial entitlements made by the government in response to societal insistence that the government assist citizens to pay for health care. Examples include Medicare and Medicaid.

Personal health care services Health care services designed to treat disease and illness, such as primary care (hospital fees, physician services).

Physical therapy assessment Identification of the altered physical (functional or structural) state that has caused activity restriction.

Practice profile Individual provider's practice patterns related to clinical outcome. Track record of efficiency and appropriate utilization of services.

Preadmission screening Requirement that tests for hospital admission be completed prior to admission.

Preferred Provider Organization (PPO) An arrangement in which a specific number of providers agree to provide services to a defined group of people at a negotiated fee-for-service rate, which is usually less than their normal rate. If the enrollee utilizes the services of a nonpreferred provider, he or she will have to pay a greater percentage of the cost of care and therefore has a greater out-of-pocket expense.

Private payers Insurance and business that assumes the major financial risk for paying for health care services.

Problem-oriented medical record (POMR) Organizational model for record keeping based on a patient problem list.

Professional liability Professional's legal responsibility or obligation to make good on any loss or damage that arises from the rendering or failure to render services to a patient or client.

Professional Review Organization (PRO) Legislative mandate with creation of Medicare and Medicaid. Its purpose is admissions review to assure quality of care and cost containment in the hospital setting. May be a physician group or a specified insurance carrier.

Prospective payment Payment made at a predetermined specific rate, on the assumption that the service can be provided for this rate. If the provider does so for less, a profit results; if not, the provider is at risk for the difference in the cost. Prospective payment originated under the Medicare amendments and are based on DRGs.

Prospective review An approval process used to determine, prior to the rendering of the care, if the proposed treatment is medically necessary and appropriate for a particular diagnosis.

Purchasers Any of a variety of entities that assume the responsibility for "buying" and "paying" for health and Workers' Compensation benefits. These entities can be PPOs, HMOs, self-insured employees, self-insured municipalities, third-party administrators.

Quality Characteristic that reflects excellence.

Quality assurance Process in which the quality of care, based on treatment standards and outcome assessment, is evaluated to determine appropriateness of care given. It is defined by JCAHO as a "process designed to objectively and systematically monitor and evaluate the quality and appropriateness of patient care, pursue opportunities to improve patient care, and resolve identified problems."

Quality management Continuous function to systematically assess and improve health care as a whole or any of its specific clinical, administrative, or support functions. Quality management includes traditional quality assurance techniques to assure minimal competence, and quality improvement techniques designed to improve the outcome of processes or interventions.

Reader   Person who reviews or uses physical therapy or medical reports to make decisions regarding some aspect of health care.

Reasonable and necessary   Set of four criteria that must be met for approval of services rendered under Medicare: (1) service is an accepted standard of medical practice and is considered to be specific and effective treatment for the condition; (2) service is at a level of complexity that requires that it be performed by a qualified physical therapist; (3) expectation that there will be improvement or potential for improvement in a reasonable length of time; (4) amount, frequency, and duration of services are reasonable.

Residual disability   Permanent restriction in performance of an activity.

Residual impairment   Permanent loss or abnormality of psychologic, physiologic, or anatomic structure or function.

Retrospective review   Review of medical care after the care has been provided, to determine if the services provided were appropriate and medically necessary. This determination is often made by review of billing statements, charts, and reports.

Retrospective fee for service   Payment of services based on actual cost of providing service. Payment is made after the service has been rendered.

Risk management   Process of planning, organizing, leading, and controlling the resources and activities of an organization to minimize the adverse effects of actual or potential accidental loss to the organization.

Second surgical opinion   Technique of prior authorization to assure that service is necessary.

Selective pricing   Predetermined setting of fees for a specific service.

SOAP   Acronym, created by Dr. Lawrence Weed that stands for subjective, objective, assessment, plan. SOAP is a daily note-writing format used with the problem-oriented medical record.

Specific task   A task can be thought of as a "piece of work" (*Webster's 9th Collegiate Dictionary*); a routine that has a specific sequence, level of accuracy, and purpose. Examples of tasks include lower-body dressing and ambulation on flat terrain.

Standard of care   Generally interpreted to mean that care given in treatment of a particular disease or injury should demonstrate the same standard ordinarily used by members of the same profession (Majority Rule).

Subsidy   Strategy used to enhance the supply of services in a health care delivery system (e.g., block grants, entitlements).

Sustainable over time   When referring to functional outcome, this term means that the level of function achieved during the course of physical therapy is maintained by the patient outside the clinical environment over a period of time.

Sustained performance   Concept used to demonstrate that the changed performance is maintained over a period of time outside the clinical environment.

Structure Measurement of qualification of staff, physical structure, licensure, and professional credentials.

Tax Equity Fiscal Reform Act (TEFRA) Act passed in 1982 and implemented in 1985 to establish requirements for the signing of Medicare-risk contracts by HMOs and competitive medical plans.

Third-party payer Claims payer that assumes responsibility for paying for health and Workers Compensation benefits without assuming any financial risk.

Two-tier system Multilevel access to health care. Usually refers to a minimal standard of care for all and higher standards for those willing and able to pay extra for care.

Utilization review Determination of whether health care services are appropriate and medically necessary on a prospective, concurrent, and/or retrospective basis, to reduce the incidence of provision of unnecessary services.

Utilization review criteria Criteria used by a reviewing party to determine whether health care services are appropriate and medically necessary.

V = Q/C Value of health care (V) is equal to its quality (Q) divided by its cost (C).

Variable premium rates When referring to menu options, an individual or employer selects a certain benefits package based on willingness to pay a specific premium based on the specific services that will be covered.

Variable work position Physical requirements of a job that allow for a variety of working postures.

APPENDIXES

Appendix I

This appendix contains the American Physical Therapy Association (APTA) Standards of Practice for Physical Therapy, Guide for Professional Conduct and Code of Ethics, and Policy Statement on Quality Assurance, by which its members abide in the practice of physical therapy. These documents are the foundation for assurance of quality physical therapy services to the public and are a guide for professional conduct in practice.

Also included are samples of reporting forms to document adverse incidents and accidents that may occur in the course of practice. These types of forms should be used in your risk management program.

I–A Standards of Practice for Physical Therapy
I–B Guide for Professional Conduct, and Code of Ethics
I–C APTA Policy Statement on Quality Assurance
I–D Incident/Accident Report

Standards of Practice for Physical Therapy*

PREAMBLE

The physical therapy profession is committed to provide an optimal level of care and to strive for excellence in practice. The House of Delegates of the American Physical Therapy Association, as the responsible body representing this profession, attests to this commitment by adopting, publishing, disseminating, and applying the following Standards of Practice. These Standards of Practice are the profession's statement of conditions and performances which are essential for quality physical therapy. They provide a foundation for assessment of physical therapy practice.

ADMINISTRATION OF PHYSICAL THERAPY SERVICE

I. Purposes and Goals
A written statement of purposes and goals exists for the physical therapy service which reflects the needs of the individuals served, the physical therapy personnel, the facility, and the community.
- Define the scope and limitation of service
- Contains current description of purpose
- List objectives and goals of services provided

*American Physical Therapy Association, Alexandria, Va., 1990.

- Is appropriate for the population (community) served
- Provides a mechanism for annual review

II. Organizational Plan

A written organizational plan exists for the physical therapy service.
- Describes the interrelationships within the overall organization
- Provides for direction of service by a physical therapist
- Defines supervisory functions within the program/service
- Reflects current personnel functions

III. Policies and Procedures

Written policies and procedures exist that reflect the operation of the service and are consistent with the purposes and goals of the physical therapy service.
- Address pertinent information about the following:
    Clinical education
    Clinical research
    Criteria for access, initiation, and termination of care
    Equipment maintenance
    Fire and disaster
    Infection control
    Job description
    Medical emergencies
    Patient care policies and protocols
    Patient rights
    Personnel-related policies
    Quality assurance
    Record keeping
    Safety
    Staff orientation
    Supervisory relationships
- Meet requirements of external agencies and state law
- Meet requirements of overall organization
- Are reviewed on a regular basis

IV. Administration

A physical therapist is responsible for the direction of the physical therapy service.
- Assures that the service is consistent with established purposes and goals
- Assures that the service is provided in accordance with established policies and procedures
- Assures compliance with local, state, and federal requirements

- Complies with current APTA Standards of Practice and Guide for Professional Conduct
- Reviews and updates policies and procedures as appropriate
- Provides appropriate education, training, and review of physical therapy support personnel

V. Staffing

The physical therapy personnel are qualified and sufficient in number to achieve the purposes and goals of the physical therapy service.

- Meet legal requirements regarding licensure and/or certification of appropriate personnel
- Provide expertise appropriate to the case mix
- Provide adequate staff-to-patient ratio
- Provide adequate support staff to professional staff

VI. Physical Setting

1. The physical setting is designed to provide a safe and effective environment that facilitates the achievement of the purposes and goals of the physical therapy service.

- Meets all applicable legal requirements for health and safety
- Meets space needs appropriate for the number and type of patients served

2. Equipment is safe and sufficient to achieve the purposes and goals of the physical therapy service.

- Meets all applicable legal requirements for health and safety
- Meets equipment needs appropriate for the number and type of patients served
- Provides for routine safety inspection of equipment by a qualified person

VII. Fiscal Affairs

Fiscal planning and management of the physical therapy service are based upon sound accounting principles.

- Include preparation and use of a budget
- Conform to legal requirements
- Are accurately recorded and reported
- Provide for optimal use of resources
- Include a plan for audit control
- Establish the basis for a fee schedule consistent with cost of service and within customary norms of what is fair and reasonable

VIII. Quality Assurance

A written plan exists for the assessment of, and action to assure, the quality and appropriateness of the physical therapy service.

- Provides for a current written plan for assessment of the service

- Provides evidence of ongoing review and evaluation of the service
- Resolves identified problems
- Is consistent with requirements of external agencies

IX. Staff Development

A written plan exists which provides for appropriate ongoing development of staff.

- Is reflected by evidence of ongoing education or attendance at continuing education activities

PROVISION OF CARE

X. Initial Evaluation

The physical therapist performs and records an initial evaluation and interprets results to determine appropriate care for the patient.

- Is initiated prior to treatment
- Is performed by the physical therapist in a timely manner
- Is documented, dated, and signed by the physical therapist who performed the evaluation
- Identifies physical therapy needs of the client
- Includes pertinent information of the following:
  History
  Diagnosis
  Problem
  Complication and precautions
  Physical status
  Functional status
  Critical behavior/mentation
  Social/environmental needs
- Provides sufficient data to establish time-related goals
- The physical therapist renders care within the scope of his or her education and experience. Appropriate referral to other practitioners is made when necessary
- The physical therapist utilizes objective measures to establish a baseline at the time of the initial evaluation
- Is documented, dated, and signed by the physical therapist who performed the evaluation

XI. Plan of Care

1. The physical therapist establishes and records a plan of care for the patient, based on the results of the evaluation.

- Includes realistic goals and expected outcome

- Is based on identified needs
- Includes effective treatment, frequency, and duration
- Recommends appropriate coordination of care with other professionals/services
- Is documented, dated, and signed by the physical therapist who established the plan of care

  2. The physical therapist involves the patient/significant other in the plan, implementation, and revision of the treatment program.
  3. The physical therapist plans for discharge of the patient, taking into consideration goal achievement, and provides for appropriate follow-up or referral.

XII. Treatment

  1. The physical therapist provides or delegates and supervises the physical therapy treatment consistent with the results of the evaluation and plan of care.

- Is under the ongoing personal care of sueprvision of the physical therapist
- Reflects that delegated responsibilities are commensurate with the qualifications of the physical therapy personnel
- Is altered in accordance with changes in individual status
- Is provided at a level consistent with current physical therapy practice

  2. The physical therapist records, on an ongoing basis, treatment rendered, progress, and change in status relative to the plan of care.

XIII. Reevaluation

The physical therapist reevaluates the patient and modifies the plan of care as indicated. The plan:

- Is performed by the physical therapist in a timely manner
- Reflects that the individual's progress is reassessed relative to initial evaluation and plan of care
- Is documented, dated, and signed by the physical therapist who performed the evaluation

EDUCATION

XIV. Professional Development

The physical therapist is responsible for his or her individual professional development and continued competence in physical therapy.

XV. Student

The physical therapist participates in the education of physical therapy students and other student health professionals

RESEARCH

XVI. The physical therapist utilizes research findings in practice, and promotes and encourages or participates in research activities.

COMMUNITY RESPONSIBILITY

XVII. The physical therapist participates in community activities to promote community health.

LEGAL/ETHICAL

XVIII. Legal
The physical therapist fulfills all the legal requirements of the jurisdictions regulating the practice of physical therapy.

XIX. Ethical
The physical therapist practices according to the Code of Ethics of the American Physical Therapy Association.

Guide for Professional Conduct*

PURPOSE

This Guide For Professional Conduct (Guide) is intended to serve physical therapists who are members of the American Physical Therapy Association (Association) in interpreting the Code of Ethics (Code) and matters of professional conduct. The Guide provides guidelines by which physical therapists may determine the propriety of their conduct. The Code and the Guide apply to all physical therapists who are Association members. These guidelines are subject to changes as the dynamics of the profession change and as new patterns of health care delivery are developed and accepted by the professional community and the public. This Guide is subject to monitoring and timely revision by the Judicial Committee of the Association.

INTERPRETING ETHICAL PRINCIPLES

The interpretations expressed in this Guide are not to be considered all-inclusive of situations that could evolve under a specific principle of the Code but reflect the opinions, decisions, and advice of the Judicial Committee. While the statements of ethical principles apply universally, specific circumstances determine their appropriate applications. Input related to current interpretations, or situations requiring interpretation, is encouraged from Association members.

*Issued by Judicial Committee, American Physical Therapy Association, October 1981. Amended January 1983, January 1984, January 1985, January 1987, January 1989, January 1991, July 1991.

Principle 1

Physical therapists respect the rights and dignity of all individuals.
1.1 Attitudes of Physical Therapists
   A. Physical therapists shall recognize that each individual is different from all other individuals and shall respect and be responsive to those differences.
   B. Physical therapists are to be guided at all times by concern for the physical, psychological, and socioeconomic welfare of those entrusted to their care.
   C. Physical therapists shall be responsive to and mutually supportive of colleagues and associates.
1.2 Confidential Information
   A. Information relating to the physical therapist–patient relationship is confidential and may not be communicated to a third party not involved in that patient's care without the prior written consent of the patient, subject to applicable law.
   B. Information derived from a component-sponsored peer review shall be held confidential by the reviewer unless written permission to release the information is obtained from the physical therapist who was reviewed.
   C. Information derived from the working relationships of physical therapists shall be held confidential by all parties.
   D. Information may be disclosed to appropriate authorities when it is necessary to protect the welfare of an individual or the community. Such disclosure shall be in accordance with applicable law.

Principle 2

Physical therapists comply with the laws and regulations governing the practice of physical therapy.
2.1 Professional Practice
   Physical therapists shall provide consultation, evaluation, treatment, and preventive care, in accordance with the laws and regulations of the jurisdiction(s) in which they practice.

Principle 3

Physical therapists accept responsibility for the exercise of sound judgment.
3.1 Acceptance of Responsibility

A. Upon accepting a patient for provision of physical therapy services, physical therapists shall assume the responsibility for evaluating that person; planning, implementing, and supervising the therapeutic program; reevaluating and changing that program; and maintaining adequate records of the case, including progress reports.

B. When the patient's needs are beyond the scope of the physical therapist's expertise, the patient shall be so informed and assisted in identifying a qualified person to provide the necessary services.

C. When physical therapists judge that benefit can no longer be obtained from their services, they shall so inform the person receiving the services. It is unethical to initiate or continue services that, in the therapist's judgment, either cannot result in beneficial outcome or are contraindicated.

D. Physical therapists shall maintain the ability to make independent judgments, which must not be limited or compromised by professional affiliations, including employment relationships.

3.2 Delegation of Responsibility

A. Physical therapists shall not delegate to a less qualified person any activity which requires the unique skill, knowledge, and judgment of the physical therapist.

B. The primary responsibility for physical therapy care rendered by supportive personnel rests with the supervising physical therapist. Adequate supervision requires, at a minimum, that a supervising physical therapist perform the following activities:

   1. Designate or establish channels of written and oral communication.

   2. Interpret available information concerning the person under care.

   3. Provide initial evaluation.

   4. Develop a plan of care, including short- and long-term goals.

   5. Select and delegate appropriate tasks of the plan of care.

   6. Assess competence of supportive personnel to perform assigned tasks.

   7. Direct and supervise supportive personnel in delegated tasks.

   8. Identify and document precautions, special problems, contraindications, goals, anticipated progress, and plans for reevaluation.

   9. Reevaluate, adjust the plan of care when necessary, perform final evaluation, and establish a follow-up plan.

3.3 Provision of Services

A. Physical therapists shall recognize the individual's freedom of

choice in selection of physical therapy services. Professional affiliations, including employment relationships, may not limit access to
services.

B. Physical therapists' professional practices and their adherence to
ethical principles of the Association shall take preference over business practices. Provisions of services for personal financial gain
rather than for the need of the individual receiving the services are
unethical.

C. Overutilization caused by continuing physical therapy services beyond the point of possible benefit or by providing services more frequently than necessary for maximum therapeutic effect is unethical.

D. If physical therapy services are misused, the physical therapist(s) involved must accept responsibility for the misuse.

3.4 Referral Relationships

A. In a referral situation where the referring source specifies the treatment program, extension of physical therapy services beyond the
proposed treatment program shall be undertaken in consultation
with the referring source.

B. Physical therapists may suggest to the referring source the possibil-
ity of referring the person under care to a qualified person whose
services may be beneficial.

C. When there is no referral, physical therapists shall refer patients under their care to other qualified persons if symptoms or conditions
are present which require services beyond the scope of their expertise or for which physical therapy is contraindicated.

3.5 Practice Arrangements

A. Participation in a business, partnership, corporation, or other entity
does not exempt the physical therapist, employer, partner or stock-
holder, either individually or collectively, from the obligation of
promoting and maintaining the ethical principles of the Association.

B. Physical therapists shall advise their employer(s) of any employer
practice which conflict with the ethical principles of the Association. Physical therapist employees shall attempt to rectify aspects
of their employment which conflict with the ethical principles of
the Association.

Principle 4

*Physical therapists maintain and promote high standards for physical
therapy practice, education, and research.*

    A. Continued Education

       Physical therapists shall participate in educational activities which enhance their basic knowledge and provide new knowledge.

    B. Whenever physical therapists provide continuing education, they shall ensure that course content, objectives, and responsibilities of the instructional faculty are accurately reflected in the promotion of the course.

4.2 Review and Self-Assessment

    A. Physical therapists shall provide for utilization review of their services.

    B. Physical therapists shall demonstrate their commitment to quality assurance by peer review and self-assessment.

4.3 Research

    A. Physical therapists shall support research activities that contribute knowledge for improved patient care.

    B. Physical therapists engaged in research shall ensure:

       1. The consent of subjects.

       2. Confidentiality of the data on individual subjects and the personal identities of the subjects.

       3. Well-being of all subjects in compliance with facility regulations and laws of the jurisdiction in which the research is conducted.

       4. The absence of fraud and plagiarism.

       5. Full disclosure of support received.

       6. Appropriate acknowledgment of individuals making a contribution to the research.

    C. Physical therapists shall report to appropriate authorities any acts in the conduct or presentation of research that appear unethical or illegal.

4.4 Education

    A. Physical therapists shall support quality education in academic and clinical settings.

    B. Physical therapists functioning in the educational role are responsible to the students, the academic institutions, and the clinical settings for promoting ethical conduct in educational activities. Whenever possible, the educator shall ensure:

       1. The rights of students in the academic and clinical setting.

       2. Appropriate confidentiality of personal information.

       3. Professional conduct toward the student during the academic and clinical educational processes.

       4. Assignment to clinical settings prepared to give the student a learning experience.

C. Clinical educators are responsible for reporting to the academic program student conduct which appears to be unethical or illegal.

Principle 5

*Physical therapists seek remuneration for their services that is deserved
and reasonable.*
5.1 Fiscally Sound Remuneration
   A. Physical therapists shall never place their own financial interest
   above the welfare of people under their care.
   B. Fees for physical therapy services should be reasonable for the service performed, considering the setting in which it is provided, practice costs in the geographic area, judgment of other organizations,
   and other relevant factors.
   C. Physical therapists should attempt to ensure that providers, agencies, or other employers adopt physical therapy fee schedules that
   are reasonable and that encourage access to necessary services.
5.2 Business Practices/Fee Arrangements
   A. Physical therapists shall not:
      1. Directly or indirectly request, receive, or participate in the di-
      viding, transferring, assigning, or rebating of an unearned fee.
      2. Profit by means of a credit or other valuable considerations, such
      as an unearned commission, discount, or gratuity in connection
      with furnishing of physical therapy services.
   B. Unless laws impose restrictions to the contrary, physical therapists
   who provide physical therapy services in a business entity may pool
   fees and moneys received. Physical therapists may divide or ap-
   portion these fees and moneys in accordance with the business
   agreement.
   C. Physical therapists may enter into agreements with organizations to
   provide physical therapy services if such agreements do not violate
   the ethical principles of the Association.
5.3 Endorsement of Equipment or Services
   A. Physical therapists shall not use influence upon patients under their
   care or their families for utilization of equipment or services based
   upon the direct or indirect financial interest of the physical therapist in such equipment or services. Realizing that these persons will
   normally rely on the physical therapists' advice, their best interest
   must always be maintained as well as their right of free choice relating to the use of any equipment or service. While it cannot be considered unethical for physical therapists to own or have a financial

interest in equipment companies or services, they must act in accordance with law and make full disclosure of their interest whenever such companies or services become the source of equipment or services for persons under their care.

B. Physical therapists may be remunerated for endorsement or advertisement of equipment or services to the lay public, physical therapists, or other health professionals provided they disclose any financial interest in the production, sale or distribution of said equipment or services.

C. In endorsing or advertising equipment or services, physical therapists shall use sound professional judgment and shall not give the appearance of Association endorsement.

Principle 6

Physical therapists provide accurate information to the consumer about the profession and about those services they provide.

6.1 Information About the Profession

Physical therapists shall endeavor to educate the public to an awareness of the physical therapy profession through such means as publication of articles and participation in seminars, lectures, and civic programs.

6.2 Information About Services

A. Information given to the public shall emphasize that individual problems cannot be treated without individualized evaluation and plans/programs of care.

B. Physical therapists may provide information about themselves to the public to facilitate the public selection of a physical therapist.

C. Physical therapists shall not use, or participate in the use of, any form of communication containing a false, plagiarized, fraudulent, misleading, deceptive, unfair, or sensational statement or claim.

D. Physical therapists shall not compensate or give anything of value to a representative of the press, radio, television, or other communication medium in anticipation of, or in return for, professional publicity in a news item.

E. A paid advertisement shall be identified as such unless it is apparent from the context that it is a paid advertisement.

Principle 7

Physical therapists accept the responsbility to protect the public and the profession from unethical, incompetent, or illegal acts.

7.1 Consumer Protection
    A. Physical therapists shall report any conduct which appears to be un-ethical, incompetent, or illegal.
    B. Physical therapists may not participate in any arrangements in which patients are exploited due to the referring sources enhancing their personal incomes as a result of referring for, prescribing, or rec-ommending physical therapy.
7.2 Disclosure
    If the physical therapist is involved in an arrangement with a referring source in which the referring source derives income from the physical therapy service, the physical therapist has an affirmative obligation to disclose to the patient that the referring practitioner derives income from the provision of the physical therapy service.

Principle 8

Physical therapists participate in efforts to address the health needs of the public.

American Physical Therapy Association Code of Ethics*

PREAMBLE

This Code of Ethics sets forth ethical principles for the physical therapy profession. Members of this profession are responsible for maintaining and promoting ethical practice. This Code of Ethics, adopted by the American Physical Therapy Association, shall be binding on physical therapists who are members of the Association.

PRINCIPLE 1

Physical therapists respect the rights and dignity of all persons.

PRINCIPLE 2

Physical therapists comply with the laws and regulations governing the practice of physical therapy.

PRINCIPLE 3

Physical therapists accept responsibility for the exercise of sound judgment.

*Adopted by the House of Delegates, June 1981. Amended June 1987, June 1991.

PRINCIPLE 4

Physical therapists maintain and promote high standards for physical therapy practice, education, and research.

PRINCIPLE 5

Physical therapists seek remuneration for their services that is deserved and reasonable.

PRINCIPLE 6

Physical therapists provide accurate information to the consumer about the profession and about those services they provide.

PRINCIPLE 7

Physical therapists accept the responsibility to protect the public and the profession from unethical, incompetent, or illegal acts.

PRINCIPLE 8

Physical therapists participate in efforts to address the health needs of the public.

APTA Policy Statement on Quality Assurance*

QUALITY ASSURANCE POLICY STATEMENT HOD 06-90-00-00

That APTA advocates voluntary member participation in quality assurance activities which are incorporated into daily practice. The commitment to quality assurance is primarily a professional responsibility and is to be promoted and fostered by Association members through individual and collective efforts. The APTA has adopted and maintained a *Guide for Professional Conduct and Code of Ethics* for the physical therapist, a *Standards of Practice for Physical Therapy* and a *Standards of Ethical Conduct for the Physical Therapist Assistant*. Each APTA chapter shall create a quality assurance committee or designate a current committee to promote quality assurance activities.

*From Quality Assurance Statement, American Physical Therapy Association House of Delegates, revised 1985, Washington, DC, 1990.

Incident/Accident Report

CONFIDENTIAL

Date of incident: _____

Persons involved:

    Staff member _____

    Staff member _____

    Patient: _____ Telephone: _____

    Visitor: _____ Telephone: _____

    Address: _____

INCIDENT/ACCIDENT:

Describe exactly: _____

    Event: _____

    Materials: _____

    Equipment: _____

    People: _____

Witnesses:

    Name: _____ Telephone: _____

    Address: _____

    Name: _____ Telephone: _____

    Address: _____

Patient's comments: _____

_____

Action: _____

_____

Date of report: _____

Report prepared by: _____

                           (Signature)

Appendix II

This appendix presents sample definitions of ICIDH (International Classification of Impairments, Disabilities, and Handicaps) codes used by policymakers to interpret the need for ongoing rehabilitation. They represent a potential method for reporting functional outcomes.

Also included in this appendix is a sample of a functional assessment tool designed by Western Neuro Care. Although numerous models are available, you may wish to develop one of your own. This guide is used to assess patient suffering from severe disability due to head injury.

An alternative impairment model that describes the sequence of decision analysis for a patient with a neurologic impairment is also presented. This model is similar to the orthopedic model presented in Chapter 3.

II–A   World Health Organization International Classification of Impairments, Disabilities, and Handicaps (Parts 40–45 and 73.0–73.8)

II–B   Neurological Impairment Model by Schenkman: Functional Disability Following Stroke

II–C   Western Physical Performance Analysis (WPPA)

II–D   Request for Therapy Services

International Classification of Impairments, Disabilities, and Handicaps*

AMBULATION DISABILITIES (40–45)*

40 Walking disability
   Includes: ambulation on flat terrain
   Excludes: negotiation of discontinuities in terrain (41–43)
41 Traversing disability
   Includes: negotiation of discontinuities in terrain such as the occasional step between different levels
   Excludes: flights of stairs (42) and other aspects of climbing (43)
42 Climbing stairs disability
   Includes: negotiation of flights of stairs and similar man-made obstacles such as ladders
   Excludes: the occasional step (41)
43 Other climbing disability
   Includes: natural obstacles
44 Running disability
45 Other ambulation disability

*Excerpted from *International Classification of Impairments, Disabilities, and Handicaps; A Manual of Classification Relating to the Cosequences of Disease.* Geneva, Switzerland, World Health Organization, 1980. Used by permission.

SKELETAL IMPAIRMENTS

Other Paralysis of Limb (73.0–73.8)

73.0 Bilateral paralysis of upper limbs
73.1 Paralysis of dominant upper limb
73.2 Other paralysis of upper limb
73.3 Bilateral paralysis of lower limbs
Excludes: paralysis classifiable to 72.3 and 72.4
73.4 Other paralysis of lower limb
73.5 Paralysis of upper and lower limbs on same side
Excludes: paralysis classifiable to 72.0, 72.1, and 72.2
73.6 Paralysis of three limbs
Excludes: paralysis classifiable to 72.5
73.7 Paralysis of all four limbs
Excludes: Paralysis classifiable to 72.6 and 72.7
73.8 Other paralysis
    73.0 Spastic paralysis, complete
    73.81 Other spastic paralysis
        Includes: spastic paresis or paralysis NOS
    73.82 Total flaccid paralysis, complete
    73.83 Other total flaccid paralysis
    73.85 Other flaccid paralysis
        Includes: flaccid paralysis NOS
    73.86 Other weakness of limbs
    73.87 Fatigue of limbs
        Excludes: fatigue NOS (94.5)

Neurologic Impairment Model

EXAMPLE OF FUNCTIONAL DISABILITY FOLLOWING STROKE

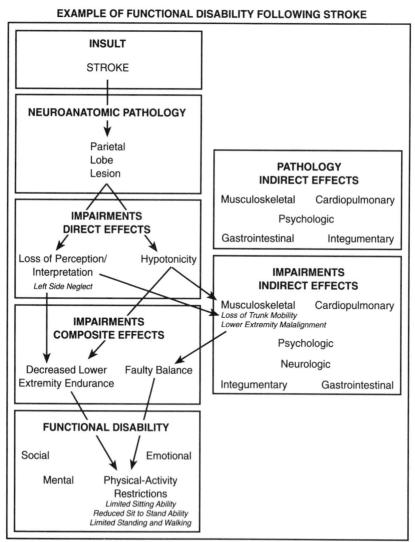

Model applied to individual who has suffered a parietal lobe lesion during a stroke. In this representation, only certain impairments related to balance and to the lower extremity are illustrated. (Adapted from Schenkman M, Butler RB: Phys Ther *July 1989, p. 541.*)

Western Physical Performance Analysis*

GUIDE TO ADMINISTERING THE WPPA

Introductory Remarks

Most, if not all, of the test positions and tasks described on the WPPA are very familiar to you as a therapist. The difference is how to *quantify* your observations. The instructions are detailed. This is to insure clear understanding across a variety of raters in various facilities.

For each task, the following order is used to improve your use of the format and accurately assess your patient's performance:

1. Test situation
2. Test behaviors (position and instruction)
3. Scoring
4. Maximizing performance

Test Situations

1. Test situations need to be as real as possible (e.g., rolling is performed in bed, dressing is assessed in the familiarity and privacy of one's room).

*Copyright © 1988, Western Neuro Care, Inc. Used by permission.

2. Test situations need to be as quiet as possible, for two important reasons: attention and privacy.
3. Test situations must reduce visual confusion. If possible, avoid creating a number of items the patient needs to scan and interpret.

Test Behaviors (Position and Instructions)

1. Always place the patient in the starting position, e.g., for rolling, the starting position is supine with the bed covers and support pillows removed.
2. Deliver test instructions *after* the patient is in the test position.
3. Limit verbal instructions to *one* sentence with the KEY WORD first. For example, say, "Roll to this side" rather than, "Now, today we are going to roll. Can you roll to the right?" Speak clearly to communicate the desired movement or task and the ending position.
4. If the patient is unable to effectively comprehend the verbal cue, then *demonstrate* or *guide* the patient through the movement. Demonstrating the movement is an alternative or complement to providing the instructions. Guiding the patient through the task is a method of maximizing the patient's performance and requires careful assessment as to the best and most appropriate score.
5. Although the WPPA is a quantitative measure, each test offers the rater an excellent opportunity to describe elements of movement pathology.

Scoring

1. Testing time
    Parts I and II: Allow 30–45 minutes
    Part III: Allow 60 minutes
2. Testing period
    Acute patient: cognitive level II or III—2 days
    Acute patient: cognitive level IV or V—1 day
    Slow-to-recover patient: cognitive levels II–VI—1 calendar week
3. Rules for the rater
    A. Rate each test by direct observation and not by recall or report.
    B. Rate each test task separately.
    C. Do not score transition from test to test (although noteworthy transition behaviors may be described elsewhere).
4. Quantitative Scores

A. Overall—Each task requires that both sides of the body be used without staff assistance or using an assistive device.

Scoring ranges from 0.0—no attempt

to 5.0—completes entire task as described.

All scores lower than 5.0 indicate that assistance or cueing is required to complete the task.

B. Specific Scores

5.0—Completes task independently.

4.0—Completes task with supervision or verbal cueing, but without physical assistance.

3.0—Completes task with minimal assistance (see key) or uses an assistance device.

2.0—Completes task with moderate assistance (see key) or minimal assistance and an assistive device.

1.0—Completes task with maximum assistance (see key).

0.0—Patient cannot, will not, or does not complete task as described OR assistance of more than one staff person is required.

C. Rating form

It is recommended that the rater use the WPPA rating form included when observing, scoring, and documenting the patient's performance.

Maximizing Performance

The WPPA attempts to score the patient's best performance. Therefore, the following steps must be taken *prior to the test procedures* to insure this outcome:

1. Patient should have sufficient time to be oriented to tasks at hand and should be given time following arousal or awakening to focus on both auditory and visual input.

2. Avoid testing when the patient is obviously fatigued. For the very low-level patient, this may mean testing only for short periods of time.

3. Patient should be fed and have sufficient time to permit food to be partially digested. For patients on nasogastric (NG) or gastric (G) tube feedings, provide time (approximately 45 minutes), following a bolus feeding.

4. Patient's airways should be clear of unusual amounts of secretions. Patients with tracheostomies may always have some secretions and cough may be stimulated when mobilizing their trunk. If this should occur, allow patient to restart the task.

5. In general, provide specific treatment to:
   - Control and prevent agitation
   - Normalize tone
   - Increase patient's attention

Within each task the developers of the WPPA and the therapy staff at Western Neuro Care have suggested types of approaches they have employed prior to testing, and which have been found useful to maximize the patient's performance.

6. Within the testing environment, the instructions provided have been designed to:
   - Limit episodes of pain
   - Limit hyperarousal
   - Limit abnormal postural reflexes

WPPA TASKS: SUPPORTED

Rolling

Test Behavior
Start: Supine in bed
Transition: Patient rolls onto side using one of several approaches.
End: Side-lying with upper limbs either lowered to bed or held with opposite limb.

Test Position
Patient is placed supine in bed with bed covers removed, and support pillows (except head pillow) removed. Bedrails are in a down position. Splint may be removed to improve ease of movement. Patient's best score, i.e., best side to roll to, is rated.

Test Instructions
Verbal: "Roll to this side." (Rater is on the desired side.)
Visual: Beckon patient to the side with hand gestures.

Maximizing Performance

1. Guide patient through rolling motion to side-lying position.
2. Use bedrails in up position to increase patient's sense of security and to guide the direction of motion.

3. Use bedrail, placing SUE on rail for patient to use.
4. Rolling is a difficult movement with which to start, therefore it may be tested during or after a treatment session or other tests.
5. Cue patient through component moves (e.g., turn head, reach with arm, lift leg). Sequence is not important for scoring purposes.

WPPA TASKS: NONSUPPORTED

Sit to Stand

Test Behavior
Start: Patient is in erect sitting position.
Transition: Patient assumes standing position by taking no more than a single step.
End: Patient is in bilateral stance with 80% erect posture (80% erect posture—the minimum amount of extension required to remain within one's base of support.).

Test Position
Patient is placed sitting at bedside with feet on floor. Patient may be assisted in achieving static sitting balance.

Test Instructions
Verbal: "Stand up" or "Stand at the side of the bed."
Visual: Sitting across from the patient, demonstrate coming to a stand from seated position.

Maximizing Performance

1. Facilitate maximum bilateral dorsiflexion.
2. Facilitate weightbearing through the ankle and forefoot.
3. Facilitate lumbar and cervical extension in sitting position.
4. Active trunk flexion.
5. Encourage the patient to utilize upper extremities.

WPPA TASKS: COMPLEX

For hygiene tasks, the location of the patient depends on the ability of the patient. Location can be in bed, on a chair, or in the bathroom.

Each patient is an individual and began these tasks prior to the injury in his/her own way. The testing therapist must be flexible enough to allow the patient to begin each task according to the patient's uniqueness. The treating therapist should inform the testing therapist of any individual differences.

Due to perceptual deficits, demonstrations of dressing tasks may be confusing to the patient. If this occurs, hand-over-hand guidance is suggested prior to the actual test episode.

Hair Combing

Test Behavior
Start: Patient supported, with brush or comb placed on the table within one-third of the patient's central visual field. The item is within the known range of the upper extremity.
Transition: Patient thoroughly combs own hair in all areas.
End: Patient completes the activity within 5 minutes.

Test Position
Same as for toothbrushing. Items required are comb or brush. Use mirror if available.

Test Instructions
Verbal: "Comb your hair" or "Brush your hair."
Visual: Imitate combing your own hair.

Maximizing Performance
Same as for toothbrushing. This also applies to hygiene and grooming tasks. Do not use mirror if the patient becomes confused.

WPPA KEY: RATING COMPLEX TASKS

5.0—Patient is given all materials and independently initiates and completes the task including, for example, wiping mouth after brushing teeth.

4.0—Requires cueing due to cognitive deficits, e.g., unable to sequence multiple steps to don a shirt.

3.0—Requires minimal assistance (<50%) to initiate, follow through, or complete the task.

2.0—Requires moderate assistance (50% effort) to complete task. If hand-over-hand guidance is needed, carryover activity is seen if guidance is stopped.

1.0—Requires maximum assistance (>50%). If hand-over-hand guidance is stopped, patient stops.

0.0—Patient is not aware of task, lacks range of motion (ROM) to perform task or refuses.

WESTERN NEURO CARE CENTER
WESTERN PHYSICAL PERFORMANCE ANALYSIS

WPPA RATING FORMS: SUPPORTED TASKS

PATIENT'S NAME: _____   DATE: _____

Indicate by circling the best score.

ROLLING
    5.0—Rolls to best side from supine without bedrails or attendant.
    4.0—Requires verbal cues.
    3.0—Requires minimal assistance (<50% effort) to initiate or complete task or uses bedrail/device.
    2.0—Requires moderate assistance (50% effort) to initiate, continue, or complete rolling, or requires assistance to use bedrail/device.
    1.0—Requires maximum assistance (>50% effort).
    0.0—Does not actively participate, or requires assistance of two or more attendants.

SUPINE TO SIT
    5.0—Comes to sitting with trunk upright, hips flexed to 90° from lying without attendant or devices.
    4.0—Requires verbal cues.
    3.0—Requires minimal assistance (<50%) to come to sit.
    2.0—Requires moderate (50%) assistance.
    1.0—Requires maximum assistance (>50%)
    0.0—Does not actively participate, lacks adequate ROM to sit, or requires assistance of two or more attendants.

SITTING BALANCE
    5.0—Sits with feet on floor, no weight on UEs, maintains head and trunk upright for 30 seconds without attendant, device, or backrest.
    4.0—Maintains sitting with verbal cues.
    3.0—Requires minimal assistance (<50% effort) *or* device.
    2.0—Requires moderate assistance (50% effort) *or* BUE support.
    1.0—Requires maximum assistance (>50%)
    0.0—Does not actively participate, or lacks ROM for sitting.

UE MOVEMENT IN SITTING
    5.0—Lifts arm(s) toward object without loss of balance.
    4.0—Requires verbal cues.
    3.0—Requires minimal assistance (<50% effort) to complete task, or requires SUE support to move the opposite UE
    2.0—Requires moderate assistance (50% effort) to complete task.
    1.0—Requires maximum assistance (>50% effort) to complete tasks.
    0.0—Does not participate, unable to attain *or maintain* sitting balance.

Scores represent the patient's ability to complete a given task.

SCORE: _____   TOTAL WPPA SCORE _____

PT/OT _____   FACILITY _____

WESTERN NEURO CARE CENTER
WESTERN PHYSICAL PERFORMANCE ANALYSIS

WPPA RATING FORMS: NONSUPPORTED TASKS

PATIENT'S NAME: _____ DATE: _____

Indicate by circling the best score.

SIT TO SIT: TRANSFERS FROM BED TO CHAIR
 5.0—Transfers from sitting bedside to chair, with feet on floor, trunk and head controlled without attendant or equipment.
 4.0—Transfers with verbal cues.
 3.0—Requires minimal (<50% effort) assistance to complete task.
 2.0—Requires moderate (50% assistance) to complete task.
 1.0—Requires maximum assistance (>50% effort) to complete task.
 0.0—Does not actively participate, lacks ROM for sitting. Requires assistance of two or more attendants, or withdraws feet from floor.

SIT TO STAND
 5.0—Comes to full upright standing from sitting without attendant and ends in stance.
 4.0—Requires verbal cues.
 3.0—Requires minimal assistance (<50% effort) to complete task.
 2.0—Requires moderate assistance (50% effort) to complete task.
 1.0—Requires maximum assistance (>50% effort) to complete task.
 0.0—Does not actively participate, or requires assistance of two or more attendants, or lacks ROM to come to standing.

STANDING BALANCE
 5.0—Standing with weight on both feet, trunk and head erect, hips and knees aligned over feet without attendant or device, and maintains for 15 minutes.
 4.0—Maintains balance with verbal cues.
 3.0—Requires minimal assistance (<50% effort) or LE device (AFO), or support of single UE.
 2.0—Requires moderate assistance (50% effort) or device and assistance.
 1.0—Requires maximum assistance (>50% effort).
 0.0—Does not actively participate, does not stand, or requires assistance of 2 or more attendants.

AMBULATION
 5.0—Initiates walking from stance, walks 15 feet without attendant and terminates in stance.
 4.0—Requires verbal cues.
 3.0—Requires minimal assistance (<50% effort).
 2.0—Requires moderate assistance (50% effort).
 1.0—Requires maximum assistance (>50% effort).
 0.0—Does not actively participate, lacks ability to stand, or requires assistance of two or more attendants.

Scores represent the patient's ability to complete a given task.

SCORE: _____ TOTAL WPPA SCORE _____

PT/OT _____ FACILITY _____

WESTERN NEURO CARE CENTER
WESTERN PHYSICAL PERFORMANCE ANALYSIS

WPPA RATING FORMS: NONSUPPORTED TASKS

PATIENT'S NAME: _____ DATE: _____

Indicate by circling the best score.

TOOTHBRUSHING
    5.0—Prepares toothbrush, brushes teeth, manages secretions in 10 minutes or less.
    4.0—Requires verbal cues only due to cognitive deficits.
    3.0—Requires minimal physical assistance (<50% effort) for initiation, preparation, or completion.
    2.0—Requires moderate physical assistance (50% effort) for initiation, preparation thoroughness during task performance. Some patient carryover is seen if hand-over-hand guidance is stopped.
    1.0—Requires maximum physical assistance (>50% effort) throughout. If hand-over-hand guidance is stopped, patient stops.
    0.0—Not aware of task, lacks ROM to perform task or refuses.

HAIR COMBING
    5.0—Given comb/brush, combs hair in 5 minutes or less.
    4.0—Requires verbal cues only due to cognitive deficits.
    3.0—Requires minimal assistance (<50% effort) for initiation, preparation, or completion of task.
    2.0—Requires moderate assistance (50% effort) for initiation, preparation, or completion of task.
    1.0—Requires maximum assistance (<50% effort) throughout. If hand-over-hand guidance stops, patient stops.
    0.0—Unaware of task, lacks ROM to perform task, or refuses.

SHIRT DONNING
    5.0—Given shirt, patient will don it completely.
    4.0—Requires verbal cues only due to cognitive deficits.
    3.0—Requires minimal physical assistance (<50% effort) for preparation, initiation, or completion.
    2.0—Requires moderate assistance (50% effort) for preparation, initiation thoroughness during task performance, and completion. If physical assistance stops, some patient carryover is seen.
    1.0—Requires maximum assistance (>50% effort) throughout. Patient is aware of task, but if physical assistance stops, patient stops.
    0.0—Patient is not aware of tasks, or refuses.

PANTS DONNING
    5.0—Given pants, patient dons pants completely.
    4.0—Requires verbal cues to perform task owing to cognitive deficits.
    3.0—Requires minimal physical assistance (<50% effort) for preparation, initiation, or completion.
    2.0—Requires moderate physical assistance (50% effort) for preparation and initiation.
    1.0—Requires maximum assistance (>50% effort).
    0.0—Patient is not aware of task, or refuses.

Scores represent the patient's ability to complete a given task.

SCORE: _____   TOTAL WPPA SCORE _____

PT/OT _____ FACILITY _____

Request for Therapy Services*

INSTRUCTIONS

For each of the following activities, please indicate how important it is to obtain care so you can improve and perform better on this activity. Following the importance rating, ask the patient and/or caregiver to prioritize the activities: "compared to all the other activities listed, how much would you like therapy with each of the following?"

RATING

1—Not at all important
2—Somewhat important
3—Moderately important
4—Very important
5—Extremely important

*From Allen C, Earhart CA: *Treatment goals for cognitive and physical disability.* Rockville, Md., American Occupational Therapy Association, in press. Used by permission.

Activity	Rating				
	1	2	3	4	5
Sitting					
Standing					
Rolling					
Moving arms					
Moving legs					
Transfer to/from bed					
Transfer to/from chair					
Transfer to/from toilet					
Toileting					
Transfer to/from shower					
Transfer to/from both					
Bathing					
Transfer to/from car					
Driving					
Walking at home					
Walking in neighborhood					
Walking in community					
Using the stairs					
Dressing					
Grooming					
Using appliances					
Using phone					
Doing laundry					
Washing dishes					
Shopping					
Managing children					
Lifting					
Carrying					
Reaching					
Stooping, squatting					
Typing					

Appendix III

This appendix presents pertinent sections from a variety of hospital manuals which should be consulted if you are providing services to Medicare patients. Also included are sample reporting forms along with instructions for completing them. These forms are included as examples and are subject to change. Consult your facility utilization review department to be sure you have the latest forms.

III–A Medicare Hospital Manual, Transmittal No. 550
III–B Medicare Skilled Nursing Facility Manual, Transmittal No. 262
III–C Medicare Skilled Nursing Facility Manual, Transmittal No. 270
III–D Medicare Intermediary Manual, Part 3 Claims Process, Transmittal 1398
III–E Plan of Care/Assessment for Outpatient Rehabilitation, Form HCFA 700
III–F Updated Plan of Care/Progress for Outpatient Rehabilitation, Form HCFA-701(9-89)
III–G Optional Updated Progress for Outpatient Rehabilitation, Form 702

APPENDIX III — A

Medicare Hospital Manual

Transmittal No. 550, August 1988

Revised Material	Revised Pages	Replaced Pages
Table of contents Chapter IV	3–76.3 (1 p)	3–76.3 (1 p)
Sec. 515	375–389 (15 pp)	

NEW PROCEDURES

Effective Date: November 11, 1988

Section 515, Billing for Part B, Outpatient Physical Therapy (OPT) Services.—This provides guidelines to use in submitting claims for outpatient PT to intermediaries. Specific guidance is provided for the type of documentation needed from you for intermediaries to perform an adequate medical review (MR). The guidelines apply to all OPT bills submitted to intermediaries. They do not apply to PT services provided under a home health plan of treatment or to PT services furnished by CORFs.

Medicare Skilled Nursing Facility Manual

Transmittal No. 262, December 1987

Revised Material	Revised Pages	Replaced Pages
Table of Contents Chapter II	2-1–204 (4 pp)	2-1–2-4 (4 pp)
Sec. 214–214.6 (cont)	2-15–23 (15 pp)	2-15–2-23 (9 pp)
Sec. 280.9	2-89–2-92 (4 pp)	1-89–2-93 (5 pp)

CHANGED IMPLEMENTING INSTRUCTIONS

Effective Date: For claims processed on or after February 1, 1988

Section 280.9, Covered Level of Care—General.—This section has been revised in its entirety for greater clarity and in order to help ensure that the guidelines are implemented in a uniform and consistent manner.

Section 280.9, Custodial Care.—This section has been revised to delete outdated and extraneous material and to provide clear examples of types of care that are considered custodial.

APPENDIX $\mathrm{III-C}$

Medicare Skilled Nursing Facility Manual

Transmittal No. 270, August 1988

Revised Material	Revised Pages	Replaced Pages
Table of Contents Chapter V	5-1–5-4 (4 pp)	5-1–50-4 (4 pp)
Sec. 542	5-25–5-6.14 (16 pp)	5-25–5-26 (2 pp)

NEW PROCEDURES

Effective Date: November 11, 1988

Section 542, Billing For Part B, Outpatient Physical Therapy (OPT).—This provides guidelines to use in submitting claims for outpatient PT to intermediaries. Specific guidance is provided for the type of documentation needed from you for intermediaries to perform adequate MR. The guidelines apply to all OPT bills submitted to intermediaries. They do not apply to PT service provided under a home health plan of treatment or to PT services furnished by CORFs.

APPENDIX III — D

Medicare Intermediary Manual
Part 3: Claims Process

Transmittal No. 1398, August 1988

Revised Material	Revised Pages	Replaced Pages
Table of Contents Chapter X	10-1 (1 p)	10-1 – 10-2 (2 pp)
Sec. 3904	10-53 – 10-69 (17 pp)	10-53 – 10-93 (41 pp)

NEW PROCEDURES

Effective Date: November 11, 1988

Section 3904, Medical Review (MR) of Part B, Intermediary Outpatient Physical Therapy (OPT) Bills.— This provides criteria to identify OPT services that must be reviewed by your MR staff. You may select these cases manually or by computer. You may review all OPT bills instead of selecting some. You may review more claims than those identified here. However, you must conform to the MR requirements for all outpatient cases identified from rehabilitation agencies, skilled nursing facilities, hospitals, and home health agencies that provide OPT in addition to home health services.

These criteria do not apply to inpatient PT services or to PT services provided under a home health plan of treatment or to PT services furnished by CORFs.

The criteria for MR case selection are based upon ECD-9-CM diagnoses, lapsed time from start of care and number of treatments (at the billing provider). See Exhibit I.

NOTE: It is prohibited to deny a bill solely on the basis that it exceeds the criteria or the diagnosis is not included in Exhibit I. (See CPEP standards, make accurate coverage determinations, S2901.4 administrative guides, Standard I.) The edits are for selecting bills to review and for paying bills that meet the edits.

Do not provide automatic coverage up to these criteria. They neither guarantee minimum coverage nor set maximum coverage limits.

Notify providers and State Physical Therapy Association chapters that you will implement these guidelines.

If more or less claims development is expected (depending upon the MR procedure selected) inform your providers. Implement the guidelines using ongoing maintenance funding. If special funding is required, notify your RO.

Plan of Care/Assessment for Outpatient Rehabilitation

(Complete for Initial Claims Only)

1. PATIENT'S LAST NAME	FIRST NAME	MIDDLE INITIAL	2. HICN

3. PROVIDER NO.	4. RESIDENCE □ SNF □ NF □ MR □ NA	5. TYPE: □ PT □ OT □ SLP □ SN □ CR □ RT □ PS □ SW

6. PRIOR THERAPY (Same Condition)
  FROM   THROUGH
	7. PRIOR HOSPITALIZATION □ NA
	  FROM TO

8. PRIMARY DX	9. SECONDARY DX

10. ONSET DATE	11. REFERRAL DATE	12. SOC. DATE

13. PRIOR LEVEL OF FUNCTION; PERTINENT HISTORY (Prior therapy results, reason for referral.)

14. INITIAL ASSESSMENT/SAFETY PRECAUTIONS/MEDICAL COMPLICATIONS (Level of function at start of care. Be specific: use objective measures, list problems.)

15. TREATMENT DX (If different from medical DX)   16. DATE OF ASSESSMENT

17. INITIAL POC (Specify procedures, modalities, short- and long-term goals.)

18. FREQ.   19. DURATION

20. FUNCTIONAL LEVEL (End of claim period)

21. DATE LAST VISIT: _____

22. SIGNATURE (or name of professional establishing POC)   23. DATE POC ESTABLISHED

24. PHYSICIAN SIGNATURE ☐ ON FILE OR ENTER HERE: _____   25. DATE: _____

I certify the need for these services furnished under this plan of care
and while under my care and if for partial hospitalization, services are
required in lieu of inpatient psychiatric care.

26. CERTIFICATION
FROM   THROUGH

INSTRUCTIONS FOR COMPLETION OF THE FORM HCFA-700 (ENTER DATES AS 6 DIGITS MONTH, DAY, YEAR)

1. Patient's Name—Enter the patient's last name, first name and middle initial.
2. HICN—Enter the patient's health insurance claim number as shown on his health insurance (Medicare card); certification award, utilization notice, temp. elig. notice, or reported by SSO.
3. Provider Number—Enter the number issued by Medicare to the billing provider.
4. Residence—Check box if the patient resides in a SNF, NF, or MR facility. Check N/A, if not applicable.
5. Type—Check the type therapy claimed. CORFs may check SN or SW for skilled nursing or social services.
6. Prior Therapy—Same Condition—Enter inclusive dates of most recent therapy for the same condition. Enter N/A or unknown, if appropriate.
7. Prior Hospitalization—Enter inclusive dates of the most recent hospitalization (1st to DC day) pertinent to the patient's current POC or condition. Use N/A or unknown, if appropriate.
8. Primary DX—Enter the medical diagnosis written resulting in the therapy disorder and related to 50% or more of the effort in the POC.
9. Secondary DX—Enter the next important medical diagnosis relating to the therapy disorder (written) resulting in less than 50% of effort in the POC.
10. Onset Date—Enter the date of the onset of the primary DX or date of the most recent exacerbation. Use 01 if exact day is unknown.
11. Referral Date—Enter the date verbal orders were received or date of the written physician referral.
12. Start of Care (SOC) Date—Enter the date services began at the billing provider (the date of the 1st Medicare billable visit).
13. Prior Level of Function: Pertinent Hx—Enter a brief narrative of the pertinent history and functional deficits. Enter prior relevant surgical procedures; outcomes of prior rehabilitation. State how function changed following an exacerbation.
14. Initial Assessment—Enter level of function on assessment. List problems. State in objective, measurable terms. Include baseline tests and interpretation, as needed. For speech reading, include audiologic results, vision status and use or status of amplification.
15. Treatment Diagnosis—Enter the treatment DX for which services

are rendered. For example for SLP, while CVA is the primary medical DX, the treatment DX might be aphasia. If same as medical DX enter SAME.

16. Date of Assessment—Enter the date your assessment was completed.

17. Initial POC—Enter the specific nature of therapy to be provided. Include specific modalities and/or procedures you plan to use. Enter the short and long-term functional (CORFs-specific rehabilitation goals) goals stated in measurable objective terms. Justify intensity, if appropriate.

18. Frequency—Enter an estimate of the frequency of treatment to be rendered (e.g., 3 × week).

19. Duration—Enter an estimate of the length of time over which the services are to be rendered and express in days, weeks, or months. If visits are to be over 1 hour long state in item 17, justify.

20. Functional Level (end of claim period)—Enter functional levels obtained at the end of the claim period compared to levels shown on initial assessment. Use objective terminology. Enter any change in functional levels related to goals.

21. Date Last Visit—Enter the date of the last visit made in this claim period.

22. Signature—The signature (or name) and professional designation of the professional who established the POC.

23. Date POC Established—Enter the date the POC was initially established.

24. Physician Signature—Enter the signature of the physician who certified the POC. Check on-file box if form is not used for certification. Enter N/A if certification is not required.

25. Date—Enter the date of physician certification, even if the on-file box is checked in #24. Enter N/A if not required.

26. Certification Period—Enter the inclusive dates of the certification period, even when the on-file box is checked in #24. Enter N/A if not required.

Public reporting burden for this collection of information is estimated to average 15 minutes per response, including the time for reviewing instructions, searching existing data sources, gathering and maintaining the data needed, and completing and reviewing the collection of information. Send comments regarding this burden estimate or any other aspect of this collection of information, including suggestions for reducing this burden, to HCFA, P.O. Box 26684, Baltimore, MD 21207; and to the Office of Information and Regulatory Affairs, Office of Management and Budget, Washington, DC 20503.

Updated Plan of Care/Progress for Outpatient Rehabilitation

(Complete for Interim to Discharge Claims. Send Photocopy of HCFA-700.)

1. PATIENT'S LAST NAME	FIRST NAME	MIDDLE INITIAL	2. HICN

3. VISITS FROM SOC	4.	INTERIM D.C. ☐ ☐	5. PROVIDER NO.

6. OTHER REHABILITATION PROVIDED
   ☐ PT ☐ OT ☐ SLP ☐ CR
   ☐ RT ☐ PS ☐ SN ☐ SW

7. CHANGED PRIMARY DIAGNOSIS ☐ NA	8. DATE OF CHANGE ☐ NA

9. CURRENT PLAN UPDATE, FUNCTIONAL GOALS (Specify procedures or modalities and dates used. Photocopy of HCFA-700 is required.)

10. CHANGED FREQUENCY - PREVIOUS   CURRENT   11. DATE CHANGE   ☐ NA

12. FUNCTIONAL LEVEL (start of claim) OR ☐ PHOTOCOPY OF PREVIOUS 701 ATTACHED (In lieu of), OR ☐ NA (2nd claim or intermediary instructs otherwise.)

13. FUNCTIONAL LEVEL (at end of billing period or when providing five or more treatments per week; update at 2 weeks and at end of claim.)

14. NO. OF VISITS THIS CLAIM _____

15. JUSTIFICATION FOR CONTINUING (or reason for DC)

16. SIGNATURE (professional establishing POC)	17. DATE

18. PHYSICIAN SIGNATURE ☐ ON FILE OR ENTER HERE: _____ 19. DATE: _____

I have reviewed this plan of care and recertify a continuing need   20. RECERTIFICATION
for services. I estimated services will be needed for   FROM   THROUGH
another _____ (days, weeks, months).

INSTRUCTIONS FOR COMPLETION OF THE FORM HCFA-701 (ENTER DATES AS 6 DIGITS: MONTH, DAY, YEAR)

1. Patient's Name—Enter the patient's last name, first name and middle initial.
2. HICN—Enter the patient's health insurance claim number as shown on his health insurance (Medicare card), certification award, utilization notice, temp. elig. notice, or reported by SSO.
3. Visits from SOC—Enter the total patient sessions completed since services were started at the billing provider for the diagnosis treated, through the last visit on this bill.
4. Interim, Discharge—Check if an interim claim or the last (discharge claim).
5. Provider No.—Enter the number issued by Medicare to the billing provider.

6. Other Rehabilitation Provided—Check the box if any of these services are being concurrently provided.
7. Changed Primary Diagnosis—If the primary diagnosis has changed from that shown on the HCFA-700, enter the change (in arabic). Check N/A, if applicable.
8. Date of Change—Enter the date the primary DX changed. Check N/A if applicable.
9. Current Plan Update, Functional Goals—Enter the current plan of care and treatment goals for the patient for *this billing period*. Enter the short-term goals to reach overall long-term goals (CORFs enter specific rehabilitation goals). Justify intensity, if appropriate.
10. Changed Frequency—Enter the previous and current frequency of visits occurred. If no change enter N/A.
11. Date—Enter the date the change in frequency of visits occurred. If no change check N/A.
12. Functional Level (start of claim)—Enter a brief objective statement of functional levels and progress reached at the start of the claim period. In lieu of summary, you may photocopy and send the prior HCFA-701. Check box. Check N/A only if intermediary instructs you not provide or if your *2nd* claim.
13. Functional Level (at end of billing period)—Enter progress made at end of claim period. Use objective terminology. Date progress when function can be consistently performed or when meaningful functional improvement is made or when regression in function occurs. Stress function, medical complication, and safety.
14. No. of Visits This Claim—Enter the total visits you made in this claim period.
15. Justification For Continuing—Enter the major reason justifying the need to continue skilled rehabilitation. Stress function, medical complication, and/or safety.
16. Signature—Enter the signature and professional designation of the professional rendering care of supervising services for this claim period.
17. Date—Enter the date of signature.
18. Physician's Signature—Enter the physician's signature who is recertifying care. Check the on-file box if the form is not used for recertification. Enter N/A if recertification is not required. Estimate need in days, weeks, or months.
19. Date—Enter the date of signature even if the on-file box is checked in #18. Enter N/A if recertification is not required.

20. Recertification—Enter the recertification inclusive dates even if the on-file box is checked in #18. Enter N/A if not required.

Public reporting burden for this collection of information is estimated to average 15 minutes per response, including the time for reviewing instructions, searching existing data sources, gathering and maintaining the data needed, and completing and reviewing the collection of information. Send comments regarding this burden estimate or any other aspect of this collection of information, including suggestions for reducing this burden, to HCFA, P.O. Box 26684, Baltimore, MD 21207; and to the Office of Information and Regulatory Affairs, Office of Management and Budget, Washington, DC 20503.

(Optional) Updated Progress for Outpatient Rehabilitation

PATIENT' LAST NAME FIRST NAME MIDDLE INITIAL	2. HICN	3. PROVIDER NO.	4. INIT ☐	INTERIM ☐	D.C. ☐

PROGRESS REPORTING (*Short-term goals/objectives continued from HCFA-700 OR 701*)

5. Goal

	6. INITIAL Measure Date: ____		7. PRIOR Remeasure Date: ____		8.CURRENT Remeasure Date: ____	
9. Measure	10. Score	11. %	10. Score	11. %	10. Score	11. %

5. Goal

	6. Measure Date: ____		7. Remeasure Date: ____		8. Remeasure Date: ____	
9. Measure	10. Score	11. %	10. Score	11. %	10. Score	11. %

5. Goal

	6. Measure Date: ____		7. Remeasure Date: ____		8. Remeasure Date: ____	
9. Measure	10. Score	11. %	10. Score	11. %	10. Score	11. %

5. Goal

	6. Measure Date: ____		7. Remeasure Date: ____		8. Remeasure Date: ____	
9. Measure	10. Score	11. %	10. Score	11. %	10. Score	11. %

5. Goal

	6. Measure Date: ____		7. Remeasure Date: ____		8. Remeasure Date: ____	
9. Measure	10. Score	11. %	10. Score	11. %	10. Score	11. %

12. INTERPRETIVE SUMMARY
(Continued from HCFA 700 or 701)

_____

_____

_____

_____

_____

_____

_____

SIGNATURE *Individual rendering care)* | 17. DATE

FORM HCFA-702 (9/89)

Appendix IV

This appendix includes a sample survey form to determine physical therapist's perceptions about quality care. Also included is the APTA Quality Assurance Model for Peer Review from APTA Standards and a listing of the Joint Commission on Accreditation of Healthcare Organizations (JCAHO) Ten-Step Process for monitoring, evaluation, and problem solving to use in developing a quality assurance program.

IV–A   Survey on Quality in Physical Therapy
IV–B   JCAHO Ten-Step Process
IV–C   Model for Peer Review/APTA Standards

Survey on Quality in Physical Therapy

In the last decade, many initiatives aiming at containing escalating healthcare costs came from industrial models of competition. Chief among these was the notion of defining the quality of the care you were providing. We are interested in seeing how physical therapists across the country view quality of care in physical therapy and what efforts they are making within their own practices to look at, monitor, and assess quality. Therefore we would like to request 7 minutes of your time to answer this brief questionnaire.

Practice Information: Yrs as a P.T. _____ Type of practice _____
Yrs in Private Practice _____ Where is your practice located _____
Number of offices _____ Approx. total number of visits/year _____
Total number of therapists _____ PT __ OT __ SP __ Other _____
Approx. total number of visits/month _____.

The following standard of rating applies to the remainder of the survey:

Strongly agree	Agree	No opinion	Disagree	Strongly Disagree
4	3	2	1	0

Answer all the following questions by circling the number that is most consistent with your opinion.

Quality Issues:

0. Quality of care is presently a significant issue in medicine 4 3 2 1 0
1. Quality of care will be more of a significant issue in medicine in the near future (5 yr). 4 3 2 1 0
2. Quality will be more of a significant issue *for my practice* in the near future (5 yr). 4 3 2 1 0
3. Quality is the degree to which the care meets the current technical state of the art. 4 3 2 1 0
4. Quality is the degree to which the care meets the standard of care in my community/region or nationally. 4 3 2 1 0
5. Quality is the degree to which the care is cost-efficient. 4 3 2 1 0
6. Quality is the degree to which the care adds to the general well-being of the patient. 4 3 2 1 0
7. Quality is the degree to which the care makes the maximum possible contribution to the reduction of lost productivity. 4 3 2 1 0
8. Quality is the degree to which the care is provided by a clinician who has participated routinely in professional development experiences. 4 3 2 1 0
9. Quality is the degree to which the care provides symptomatic relief to the patient. 4 3 2 1 0
10. Quality is the degree to which the care effects complete resolution of the objective findings. 4 3 2 1 0
11. Quality is the degree to which the care meets or exceeds patient expectations for the treatment. 4 3 2 1 0
12. Quality is the degree to which the care generates referral source satisfaction. 4 3 2 1 0
13. Quality is the degree to which the care generates payer satisfaction. 4 3 2 1 0
14. Quality is the degree to which the care generates employer satisfaction. 4 3 2 1 0
15. Quality is the degree to which the care generates patient satisfaction. 4 3 2 1 0
16. Quality is the degree to which the care meets key customer satisfaction issues for the patient. 4 3 2 1 0
17. Quality is the degree to which the care leads to improved clinical outcome. 4 3 2 1 0
18. Quality is the degree to which the care generates therapist or staff satisfaction. 4 3 2 1 0
19. Quality is the degree to which the care leads to a quantifiable functional improvement. 4 3 2 1 0

20. Quality is the degree to which the care is appropriately and completely documented.   4 3 2 1 0
21. Quality is the degree to which the care leads to quantifiable functional improvement within the limits of reimbursement.   4 3 2 1 0
22. Quality is the degree to which the care is provided by the same therapist or practitioner.   4 3 2 1 0
23. Quality is the degree to which the care lowers the total work days lost due to an injury or illness.   4 3 2 1 0
24. Quality is the degree to which the care generally improves the health status of the patient.   4 3 2 1 0
25. Quality is the degree to which the care leads to a maximum improved clinical outcome within a minimum number of visits.   4 3 2 1 0
26. It is important in my practice to routinely monitor quality. 4 3 2 1 0
27. It is important in my practice to measure quality.   4 3 2 1 0
28. It is important in my practice to motivate my staff either monetarily or in other ways.   4 3 2 1 0
29. It is or will be important to motivate my staff to produce a certain *quality* of work every day or every week.   4 3 2 1 0
30. It is or will be important to motivate my staff to produce a certain *quantity* of work every day or every week.   4 3 2 1 0
31. My practice routinely *measures* quality.   4 3 2 1 0
32. My practice routinely *monitors* quality.   4 3 2 1 0
33. My practice is using incentive systems for our staff.   4 3 2 1 0
34. My practice is using incentive systems for our staff to produce a certain quantity of work every day or every week.   4 3 2 1 0
35. My practice is using incentive systems for our staff to produce a certain quality of work every day or every week.   4 3 2 1 0
36. Quality is the degree to which the care leads to a maximum improved clinical outcome within a minimum number of visits.   4 3 2 1 0

Thank you very much for your assistance! We are testing this document and would welcome any comments that may assist us in improving it. Was it difficult for you to understand? Should the information be modified? Which questions do you feel were particularly important?_____
_____
Thank you for your time.

JCAHO 10-Step Process

The 10-step process for monitoring, evaluation, and problem solving is designed to help an organization effectively use its resources to manage the quality of care provided.

Step 1: Assign responsibility
Step 2: Delineate scope of care
Step 3: Identify important aspects of care
Step 4: Identify indicators
Step 5: Set thresholds for evaluation
Step 6: Collect and organize data
Step 7: Evaluate care
Step 8: Take action; solve problems
Step 9: Assess actions; document improvement
Step 10: Communicate information to quality assurance program

For further information about the JCAHO's 10-Step Process, review The Joint Commission *Accreditation Manual for Hospitals*, 1991.

Model for Peer Review/APTA Standards

Criteria	Yes	No	Comment

Initial Evaluation
  1. Is initiated prior to treatment
  2. Is performed by the PT and is timely
  3. Is documented, dated, with legal signature of PT
  4. Includes pertinent information:
      Medical history
      Diagnosis
      Problem
      Complication/precautions
      Physical status
      Functional status
      Critical behavior/mentation
      Social/environmental
  5. Defines goals
Plan of Care
  1. Is based on identified needs
  2. Includes Rx method, frequency, and duration
  3. Documentation: coordinates care with other professionals/services
  4. Reflects involvement of family/community, etc.
  5. Anticipates discharge, includes:
      Social/environmental needs
      Outside referrals
      Community Resources
      Recommended follow-up
      Expected outcome in relationship to initial evaluation
      Expected disposition
      Home program

Criteria	Yes	No	Comment

Treatment
1. Is provided in accordance with findings
2. Is under the ongoing supervision of the PT
3. Reflects that delegated responsibilities are commensurate with the qualifications of the PT
4. Is altered in accordance with PT's change or individual status

Reevaluation
1. Reflects that the individual's progress is reevaluated to the initial evaluation and plan of care.
2. Is performed, dated, and signed by PT

Index

A

Accident report, 241
Activities of daily living (ADL) skills, 83, 86
Administrative law judge review for medicaid appeal, 161–162
Adverse incidents
documentation of, 69–70
and risk management, 69
Algorithm in documentation review, 59
American Physical Therapy Association (APTA)
Code of Ethics in, 238–239
Guide for Professional Conduct, 230–237
model definition of physical therapy, 51
model for peer review, 280–281
position on quality assurance, 66, 189–194, 240
Risk Management Resource Guide, 69
Standards of Practice, 65–66
administration of physical therapy service, 224–227
community responsibility, 229
education, 228
expert witness use of, 65–66
legal/ethical, 229
provision of care, 227–228
research, 229

Americans with Disabilities Act (ADA) (1990), 101–102, 116
APTA. *See* American Physical Therapy Association (APTA)

B

Biofeedback, medicare coverage of, 140
Business records, medical records as, 54–62

C

Certificate of Need process (CON), 15
Clinical decision-making model
applying, 86–88
case study
history of present problem, 88–89
initial physical therapy examination, 89–93
model of, 82–86
rationale for, 81–82
Clinician impression, identifying, in functional assessment, 116–118
Commission on Accreditation of Rehabilitation Facilities (CARF), in assessing quality, 191–194
Community standards, in influencing reimbursement policies, 24

Competition, health care policy focus on, 4

Competitive marketing, prospective pricing in, 15

Concurrent review of physical therapy claims, 58

Control and health care delivery system, 10, 14–16

Co-payments, 17–18

Corrected incentives, in controlling health care costs, 15

Cost containment, and health delivery, 24

Cost control
  and health maintenance organizations, 21–22
  and prospective payment, 21–22
  and rationing methods, 21–22

D

Deductibles, 17–18

Design defects in health care system, 7

Diagnosis
  basing treatment on identifying problem in, 49
  demonstration of therapist's capability in dealing with, 51–54
  importance of stating problem in, 47–48
  providing timeline for achieving functional outcome, 49–51

Diagnosis related groups (DRGs), 5

Discounted rates, 15

Documentation. *See also* Functional outcome report
  of adverse incidents, 69–70
  building, with clinical decision making model, 81–94
    applying, 86–88
    case study, 88–93
    model of orthopedic dysfunction in, 82–86
    rationale for, 81–82
  contents of ideal interim report, 44
  contents of initial report, 44
  factors to be covered in, 39–42
  identifying readers of, and relating to, 37–42
  importance of, to patient care reimbursement, 32–72
  legal considerations in, 63–70
  need for completeness in, 67–68
  need for concise style in, 67–68
  need to show effectiveness of service in, 37
  reimbursement considerations in, 44–62
    importance of stating clearly problem/diagnosis, 47–48
    translating complex professional concepts into easily understood form and language, 45
  strategies in writing, 68
  tips in writing, 42–44, 68–69
  in utilization review, 5–6

E

Economic indicators, and use of subsidies in health care systems, 11

Economics, 4

Efficiency in providing health care services, 8

Employee-based approach to health care reform, 22

Ethics
  American Physical Therapy Association code of, 238–239
  Guide for Professional Conduct in, 230–237
  Standards of Practice for Physical Therapy, 224–229
    administration of physical therapy service, 224–227
    community responsibility, 229
    education, 228
    legal/ethical, 229
    provision of care, 227–228
    research, 229

Expert witness, testimony of, 65–66

F

Functional disability, 83

Functional limitations
  definition of, 83
  identifying and reporting in functional outcome assessment, 112–116
  translating to treatment, 46–47

Functional outcome assessment, 6, 113–114
  application to Medicare documentation, 135–162
  defining activities for, 106
  identifying goals in, 120–121
  identifying and reporting in, 112–113
  in managed care, 21–22

as measure of health care value, 21–22
providing timeline for achieving, 49–51
Western physical performance analysis,
    247–255
Functional outcome report (FOR),
    121–123
  basis for, 117–118
  criteria for, 106
  evolution of reporting practices,
    103–106
  shift to more comprehensiveness in
    reporting, 101–102
  step-by-step method to, 107, 108–109
    analyzing patient performance,
      112–116
    devising treatment strategy, 121–122
    establishing patient needs, 109–112
    identifying clinician impression,
      116–118
    postulating relationships between
      impairments and performance,
      118–119
    predicting functional outcome,
      120–121
  sustained-performance model in,
    121–123
  as working process, 106–108

G

Gatekeeping, 16
Government-based approach to health care
    reform, 22
Gross National Product (GNP) and health
    care costs, 12

H

Handicap, 86
Health care, 8
  attempts to control costs of, 21
  balancing supply and demand in, 9
  causes of cost escalation, 6–7
  comparison of systems, 20–21
  defects in, as catalyst for change, 8
  distribution of expenses for, 13, 14
  efficiency in providing, 8
  escalation of costs of, 36
  flow of funds for payment of, 4
  growth in costs, 11–12
  physical therapist concern with costs of,
    23–24

public value of, 24
rationing of, 24
reasons for increasing costs, 15
reforms in, 22
reimbursement for, 8
role of physical therapist in providing,
    2–6
Health care delivery system
  coping with managed, 6–7
  market dynamics of, 5
  objectives and strategies of, 9–10
  purpose of, 7–8
  two-tier, 19
Health care policy
  evolution of U.S., 10–18
  future of, 19–25
  major views of, 5
  reforms in, 3
Health care reforms, approaches to, 22
Health Insurance Manual (HIM), 137
Health maintenance organizations (HMOs),
    15, 17
  and cost control, 21
  growth of, 8
  Medicare use of, 15, 16
Health Systems Agency (HSA), 15
Hill Burton grants, 11
Household share of health care
    expenditures, 14

I

ICD-9 code in developing provider
    profiles, 60
ICIDH. *See* International Classification of
    Impairments, Disabilities, and
    Handicaps (ICIDH)
Impairment, 83, 116–117
Incident/accident report, 241
In-person hearing for Medicaid appeal,
    161
Insurance and health care delivery, 17–18
Insurance claims representatives,
    perspectives of, on physical
    therapists, 35
Insurance industry
  and development of medically based
    criteria for payment decisions,
    104–105
  flagging of charts in evaluation of
    medical necessities, 57–58
  use of registered nurse as medical
    reviewer in, 57

International Classification of
Impairments, Disabilities, and
Handicaps (ICIDH) system, 244–246
relationship to physical therapy
reporting, 117

J

Joint Commission on Accreditation of
Healthcare Organizations (JCAHO)
agenda for changes in assessing quality,
190–191
10-step process in, 279

L

Legal considerations, in documentation,
63–70
Linear progression, 49
Locality rule in interpreting standard of
care, 65

M

Majority rule in interpreting standard of
care, 65
Malpractice
definition of, 64
major elements in, 64–65
negligence in, 64
Managed care
coping with, 6–9
and health care delivery, 24
impact of, on physical therapy, 2, 17
outcome assessments skills in, 21–22
Market dynamics of health care delivery
system, 5
Medicaid, 12
Medical impairment model in SOAP
reporting format, 117–118
Medical record
admissibility in court, 67
as business records, 54–62
problem-oriented, 103
Medicare, 12, 15
appeal process, 157, 159–162
hearing process, 160–162
Medicare Part A, 159
Medicare Part B, 159–160
carriers, 136
conditions of reasonable and necessary
care, 139–141
coverage of, 137

criteria for eligibility for physical
therapy services, 139
discharge summary, 154–157
case study, 155
critiquing, 156–157
evaluation, 141–142
assessment of findings, 143–145
case study, 147–149
critiquing, 149–150
one-time consultation, 146–147
pertinent medical history, 142
previous functional level, 142–143
reason for referral, 142
treatment of plan and goals, 145–146
health maintenance organizations use of,
15, 16
hospital manual, 260
initial evaluation case study, 166–168
intermediaries, 136
intermediary manual Part 3: claims
process, 263–264
Medicare Part A, 136–137, 138
Medicare Part B, 136–137, 139
monthly summary, 150–154
case study, 151–152, 168–170
critiquing, 154
purpose of, 135–137
skilled nursing facility manual, 261, 262
Medicare hospital manual, 260
Menu options in benefit selection process,
18

N

Negligence and malpractice claims, 64
Negotiated fees, 15
Neurologic dysfunction, practice case
study, 128
Noncovered service, 157
claims for, 157
defined, 157

O

On-the-record hearing for Medicaid
appeal, 161
Optimal health status, maintenance of, 7
Orthopedic dysfunction, 127–128
model of, 82–86
practice case study, 127–128
Outcome management, 36–37
Outpatient rehabilitation
plan of care/assessment for, 265–268

updated plan of care/progress for, 269–272
updated progress for, 273–274

P

Patient care reimbursement, importance of documentation to, 32–72
Patient needs, establishing, in functional outcome report, 109–112
Patient performance, analyzing in functional outcome assessment, 112–116
Payment subsidies in health care delivery system, 12, 14
Peer review
    model for, 280–281
    and quality assurance, 189–194
Personal health care services, 7–8
Physical therapist
    code of ethics for, 238–239
    concern with health care costs, 23–24
    Guide for Professional Conduct for, 230–237
    impact of Americans with Disabilities Act on, 101–102
    impact of managed care on, 2, 17
    motivations of, 2
    need for change in mindset, 24–25
    need to improve documentation, 35–36
    and need to understand health care delivery system, 1–6
    others' perspectives of, 35
    patient interactions with, 46
    position of professional, on quality assurance, 189–194
    as provider of health care, 2–6
    rewards of being, 25
    standards of care employed by, 65–66
Physical therapy
    APTA standards of practice for, 224–229
    carrier valuation of, 24
    changes in practice of, 104
    conditions of reasonable and necessary care, 139–141
    criteria for, 139
    evaluation of services offered by, 33–36
    identifying readers of, and relating to, 37–42
    model definition of, 51
    plan of care/assessment for outpatient rehabilitation, 265–268

quality care in, 33–35
    request for, 256–257
    survey on quality in, 276–278
    updated plan of care/progress for outpatient rehabilitation, 269–272
    updated progress for outpatient rehabilitation, 274
Physical therapy assessment, formulating, 116–118
Physical therapy reports. *See also* Documentation; Functional outcome report
    relationship between ICIDH classification system and, 117
Physician Training Capitation and Allied Health grants, 11
Practice profiles in health care delivery, 19
Preadmission screenings, 17–18
Preferred provider organizations (PPOs), 15, 17
Private market approach to health care reform, 22
Private payers, 17–18
Private sector agenda, in health care delivery, 17–18
Problems
    demonstration of therapist's capability in dealing with, 51–54
    importance of stating, in diagnosis, 47–48
    basing treatment on identifying problem, 49
    providing timeline for achieving functional outcome, 49–51
Problem-Oriented Medical Record (POMR), 103
Professional liability claims, legal considerations in, 63–70
Professional services, costs of other, 22, 23
Program evaluation, in assessing quality, 191–194
Prospective payment concept (DRGs), 5
    in competitive marketing, 15
    and cost control, 21, 22
    incentives for efficiency through, 16–17
    market-based strategies, 22
Prospective review of physical therapy claims, 58
Provider profiles in documentation review, 59–62
Purchasers, concern of, over health care costs, 36

Q

Quality
  comparison of quality assurance and
    quality improvement, 185–189
  definition of, 175–177
  JCAHO 10-step process, 279
  model for review/APTA standards,
    280–281
  survey on, in physical therapy, 276–278
Quality assurance, 5–6
  APTA policy statement on, 240
  position of physical therapists on,
    189–194
  self assessment, 194–195
    analyze key problems/opportunities
      for improvement, 202
    developing solutions, 202
    identifying problems, 195–201
    implementing and monitoring,
      203–204
    selecting and defining the highest
      priority problems opportunities for
      improvement, 201–202
Quality care
  appropriateness, 181–183
    execution, 183–184
    purpose, 184–185
  efficacy, 180–181
  high-priority elements of, 176, 180
  methods of looking at, 177–179
  in physical therapy, 33–35
  questions reflecting definitions of
    quality, 175–177

R

Rationing methods, and cost control, 21
Referral, reporting reason for, in functional
    outcome report, 109–112
Registered nurse, as medical reviewer, 57
Rehabilitation. *See* Outpatient
    rehabilitation; Patient care
    reimbursement
Reimbursement considerations
  in documentation, 44–62
    importance of clearly stating
      problem/diagnosis in, 47–48
    translating complex professional
      concepts into easily understood
      form and language, 45–47
Residual disabilities, inclusion of, in
    functional outcome report, 110–111

Residual impairments, inclusion of, in
    functional outcome report, 110–111
Retrospective fee for service, 8
Retrospective review of physical therapy
    claims, 58
Risk management, 241
  in documentation, 69–70

S

Second surgical opinions, 17–18
Selective pricing, 5
Skilled physical therapy, 137–141
SOAP (subjective, objective, assessment,
    and plant) format, 103, 117–118
Standard of care, breach of, in malpractice
    claim, 65
Standards of practice, correlation of
    documentation with, 58
Subsidies in health care delivery system,
    10–14
Sustained performance, showing in
    functional outcome reports,
    121–123

T

Tax Equity Fiscal Reform Act (1982), 16
Technician, as medical reviewer, 57
Telephone hearing for medicaid appeal,
    161
Test-retest, 121–123
Total quality management (TQM), 185
Treatment
  basing on identification problem, 49
  use of documentation in demonstrating
    efficiency of, 51–54
Treatment plan
  development of, in functional outcome
    assessment, 120–121
  providing timetable in, 49–51
Two-tier system of health care delivery, 19

U

U.S. Health Care Delivery Systems,
    importance of understanding, 1–6
Utilization review, 5–6
  in documentation, 44
  use of medical records by, 54–62
Utilization review nurses, perspectives of,
    on physical therapists, 35

Utilization review physician, as medical
reviewer, 57

V

Variable premium rates, 17–18

W

Western Physical Performance Analysis
(WPPA), 114, 247–255

Win-win situations, physical therapists
support for, 37
Workers Compensation, review of
documentation by, 58
Workers compensation companies, use of,
as medical reviewer, 57
World Health Organization. *See*
International Classification of
Impairments, Disabilities, and
Handicaps